Dr. Sebi's Approved Encyclopedia for Alkaline Herbal Remedies

100% Natural Self-Healing Guide for Erectile Dysfunction, Genital Herpes, Infertility, Endometriosis, High Blood Pressure, Heart Attack, Diabetes, Skin Diseases, Lupus, Autoimmune Diseases, Cancer, Anemia, etc.

CLEMENT JACOB

Introduction

Have you been trying so hard to get pregnant and become a mother that you have spent too much money buying and consuming ineffective and expensive drugs to treat female reproductive system disorders such as fibroids, infertility, endometriosis, abnormal uterine bleeding, PCOS, POI, cervical cancer, interstitial cystitis, etc., without getting your desired result?

Are you tired of buying and using expensive and ineffective creams, skin solutions, and supplements to treat different types of skin diseases without getting your desired result?

Are you suffering from any form of erectile dysfunction such as; infertility, premature ejaculation, low sperm count, weak erection, etc. that you have suffered countless nagging from your woman that you can't satisfy her sexual needs?

Are you or any of your loved ones suffering from chronic diseases such as; cancer, anemia, thyroid disorder, heart failure, high blood pressure, diabetes, or under dialysis…

Unlock the secrets of 100% natural, self-healing power with the Dr. sebi's approved encyclopedia for alkaline herbal remedies In this guide, you will learn how to use Dr. Sebi's time-tested, alkaline methodology "The 2 steps of healing methodology" with alkaline diets and spring water to rid the body of chronic conditions. From erectile dysfunction and infertility to diabetes, autoimmune disorders, and cancer, this comprehensive guide provides healing insights for over a dozen health conditions using only natural herbs and alkaline diets.

In this book, the author features Dr. Sebi's nutritional guide, a full list of approved herbal teas, and over 70 alkaline herbs specifically chosen to detoxify, energize, and restore the body to its original alkaline state where diseases cannot survive. This encyclopedia is the bridge between ancient wisdom with modern health needs. Whether you want to revitalize your body, manage persistent ailments, or embrace a naturally balanced lifestyle, this book got you covered as it empowers you to take control of your well-being and achieve true, lasting health.

Contents

CHAPTER ONE
Dr. Sebi's Approved Nutritional Guide
Approved Vegetables

The vegetables approved by the late Dr. Sebi are:

1. Amaranth green (same as callaloo, a green variety)

2. Cucumber

3. Avocado

4. Kale

5. Lettuce (All except icebag)

6. Izote (Cactus flower or leaf)

7. Bell pepper

8. Dandelion green

9. Garbanzo beans

10. Mushrooms (All except shitake)

11.   Okra

12.   Zucchini

13.   Green Banana

14.   Onions

15.   Chayote (Mexican Squash)

16.   Olives

17.   Poke Salad (Green)

18.   Tomato (Cherry and plum only)

19.   Squash

20.   Watercress

21.   Purselane (Verdolaga)

22.   Tomatilo

23.   Sea   Vegetable
        (Arame/Wakame/Dulse/Nort)

24.   Turnip Greens

25.   Nopales (Mexican Cactus)

Approved Fruits
The fruits approved by the late Dr. Sebi are:

1. Mango

2. Apples

3. Bananas (Smallest one or the burro/midsize)

4. Tamarind

5. Prunes

6. Plums

7. Papaya

8. Melons (Seeded)

9. Berries (All types of elderberries except cranberries)

10.   Orange (Seville or sour)

11.   Prickly pear (Cactus fruit)

12.   Limes (Key limes with seed)

13.   Cantaloupe

14.   Currants

15.   Peaches

16.   Pears

17.   Chirimoya (Sugar apple)

18.   Raising (Seeded)

19.   Soursops (West Indian or Latin markets)

20.   Dates

21.   Soft Jelly coconuts

22.   Figs

23.   Grapes

24.   Cherries

Approved Grain

The grains approved by the late Dr. Sebi are:

1. Kamut

2. Spelt

3. Rye

4. Teff

5. Wild rice

6. Quinoa

7. Fonio

8. Amaranth

Approved Herbal Teas

The natural herbal teas recommended by the late Dr. Sebi are:

1. Ginger

2. Tila

3. Burdock

4. Elderberry

5. Anise

6. Fennel

7. Raspberry

8. Allspice

9. Chamomile

10. Cuachalalate

11. Muicle

12. Gordo Lobo

13. Flor de Manita

14. Burdock

Approved Nuts and Seeds

The nuts and seeds recommended by the late Dr. Sebi are:

1. Brazilian nuts

2. Raw Sesame "Tahini"

3. Raw sesame seeds

4. Walnuts

5. Hemp seeds

Approved Oils

The oils recommended by the late Dr. Sebi are:

1. Avocado oil

2. Sesame oil

3. Olive oil (Not cooked)

4. Coconut oil (Not cooked)

5. Hemp seed oil

6. Grapeseed oil

Approved Spices and Seasoning

The spices and reasoning recommended by Dr. Sebi

are categorized into four (mid-flavors, pungent spicy flavor, salty flavor, and Sweet flavor).

Mid-flavors: The mid-flavors are:

1. Basil

2. Thyme

3. Bay leaf

4. Tarragon

5. Cloves

6. Sweet Basil

7. Dill

8. Savory

9. Parsley

10. Oregano

The pungent and spicy flavor are:

1. Sage

2. Achiote

3. Habanero

4. Cayenne (African Bird Pepper)

5. Onion Powder

6. Coriander (Cilantro)

Salty flavor: The salty flavors recommended by the late Dr. Sebi are:

1. Pure sea salt

2. Powdered granulated seaweed (kelp)

Sweet flavor: The sweet flavors recommended by the late Dr. Sebi are:

1. Date sugar

2. Pure agave syrup

Does and Don't of Late Dr. Sebi During and After Cleansing

The does and don'ts of late Dr. Sebi during and after cleansings are:

1. Make sure you consume only the food that are listed in Dr. Sebi's nutritional guide

2. Drink at least a gallon of natural spring water daily

3. Avoid the consumption of diary product, animal product and fish.

4. Avoid the consumption of alcohol 100%

5. Avoid the consumption of hybrid food.

6. Avoid the consumption of food that is microwaved 100%.

7. Avoid the consumption of seedless fruit.

8. Avoid the consumption of canned and other chemical preserved foods

9. It's of a great benefit to cleanse at least once a year for seven days, if you are consuming an alkaline whole food plant based diet. If you do not maintain a whole food plant based diet, it is recommended that you cleanse for at least 7 days after every three months. keep in mind that consuming foods that are acidic to the body will put the body at risk of relapsing.

CHAPTER TWO
Approved Herbs
The list of herbs approved by the late Dr. Sebi are:

1. Nopal

2. Huereque/Wereke

3. Muicle (Mexican Honeysuckle)

4. Locust Bark (Black Locust)

5. Marula

6. Hawthorn Berry

7. Arnica

8. Lupulo

9. Lily of the Valley

10.   Manzo (Yerba Del Manzo)

11.   Eyebright

12.   Kelp plant

13.   Cordoncillo Negro

14.   Red Raspberry leaves

15.   Shepherd's purse

16.   Peony

17.   Horsetail/Shavegrass

18.   Black Walnut

19.   Draco (Dragon's blood)

20.   Juniper berry

21.   Blessed Thistle

22.   German Chamomile

23.   Hierba Del Sapo (Eryngium)

24.   Stinging Nettle

25.   Bitter Melon

26.   Conconsa/Cancansa

27.   Blue Vervain

28.   Batana Oil

29.   Bugleweed

30.   Burdock Root

31.   Eucalyptus

32.   Flor De Manita

33.   Irish Sea Moss

34.   Gordolobo (Great Mullein),

35.   Capadulla

36.   Flor De Tila

37.   Bladderwrack

38.   Chickweed

39.   Condurango

40.   Rhubarb Root

41. Cascara Sagrada

42. Anamu/Guinea Hen Weed

43. Dandelion

44. Chamomile

45. Cocolmeca

46. Chaparral

47. Yarrow

48. Sarsaparilla Root

49. Hydrangea

50. Valerian Root

51. Pavana

52. Kalawalla

53. Gingsen

54. Contribo

55.   Cuachalalate

56.   Chaparro Amargo

57.   Damiana

58.   Elderberry (Black)

59.   Hombre Grande

60.   Fennel

61.   Palo Guaco

62.   Pao Pereira

63.   Palo Mulato

64.   Cablote

65.   Linden

66.   Sage

67.   Prodigiosa

68.   Red Clover

69.   Tilia (Linden)

70.   Tronadora

71.   Yellow Dock (Root)

72.   Valerian

73.   Yohimbe Bark (Yohimbi)

74.   Pygeum

75.   Cilantro

76.   Olive leaf

77.   Holy Basil

78.   Pau d'Arco

CHAPTER THREE
Five Ways to Detoxify/Cleanse the Body System (Intra-cellular Cleansing)
What Is Detoxification?

Detoxification is a holistic wellness practice designed to cleanse the body of harmful toxins (unwanted substances) that accumulate over time and have the potential to affect health negatively in the long run. Late Dr. Sebi's detox methods focus on supporting the body's natural processes through dietary adjustments, spring water consumption, and using natural herbs to reverse the body back to its original alkaline state, boost energy levels, improve digestion, and enhance overall well-being.

A detox can be done in several ways, and the most common type of detox is fasting. There are various fasts, including:

1. Water fast

2. Liquid fast

3. Smoothie fast

4. Fruit fast

5. Raw food fest

1. Water fast: Water fast is only consuming water throughout the number of days that you have decided to do a detox. (Spring water)

2. Liquid fast: A liquid fast involves consuming water and juices. These can include fruit and vegetable juices and herbal teas.

3. Smoothie fast: Smoothie fast is consuming only smoothies that contain fruits and sometimes vegetables that are approved by the late Dr. Sebi (DR. Sebi's nutritional guide)

4. Fruit fast: A fruit fast involves eating only the fruits approved in Dr. Sebi's nutritional guide and, of course, spring water.

5. Raw food fast: A raw food fast involves eating

raw fruits and vegetables from Dr. Sebi's nutritional guide.

Please note that any of these types of fasts can be done as a form of detoxing or cleansing, or there can be a combination depending on the fasting method that you choose. You might want to focus on only consuming the drinks and foods that are specific to your cleansing needs, and the cleansing herbs are highly recommended while detoxing because they will accelerate the healing process.

This is done by eliminating toxins through the body faster than normal because, without the cleansing herbs, it can cause more side effects and symptoms.

What Is the Best Duration to Do a Detox?

The best duration for a detox depends on the individual's tolerance and level of toxins. Typically, it is recommended to detox for 7 to 14 days, however, some people detox for 30 to 90 days. If you have health issues that make it difficult for you to fast on water or juice, I recommend fasting on fruits and or raw veggies approved by Dr. Sebi (fruits and veggies listed in Dr. Sebi's nutritional guide). Irrespective of the type of fast you decide to embark on, you will still get results, but it may take a little longer. Therefore, I recommend you do a cleanse for at least 90 days for such type of fast.

Is There Any Symptoms During Detox?

Yes, there are some common symptoms which include:

1. Feeling cold

2. A hard time sleeping or sleeplessness

3. Cold and flu symptoms

4. Tongue discoloration

5. Itching and rashes

6. Aches and pains

7. Changes in bowel movements

8. Low energy

9. Outbreaks

10.   Expelling excess mucus

11.   Low blood pressure, etc.

Please do not panic when you experience any of the above symptoms as all the symptoms are temporary and usually subside after the first week.

When Do I Need to Start the Revitalization?

Revitalizing is recommended immediately after cleansing. Irrespective of the number of days that you fast, whether it is a week or one month you will still benefit from the cleanse. Remember that the amount of time that you cleanse greatly helps with the healing process, but it is not the only factor. Detoxing for a longer period usually yields better results than a shorter period. However, once you have started the water or liquid fast for the first three days, the digestive tract will start to slow down. This will allow the body to focus more energy on healing the body because it is no longer using energy to digest food. If you are on a water or liquid fast, it is of great importance to gradually reintroduce solid foods back into your system. It is recommended that you consume fruit that has high levels of water, such as watermelon and berries, 3 days before you finish your fast. For example, if you are fasting on water or liquid for 14 days, on the 12th day, you should introduce watermelon and berries. On the 13th day, you can introduce cucumber, bananas, and apples while slowly reintroducing vegetables and solid foods on the 15th day.

Please note that, if you have fasted on fruit and or raw veggies you can skip this step.

CHAPTER FOUR
Herbal Remedy for Erectile Dysfunction
The Cleansing Herbs for Erectile Dysfunction (ED)

The cleansing herbs for erectile dysfunction (ED) such as low sperm count, weak erections, premature ejaculation, poor sexual performance, low libido, low energy, and stamina level, etc. are:

1. Burdock Root

2. Cascara Sagrada

3. Chaparral

4. Dandelion

5. Elderberry

6. Mullein

7. Eucalyptus

8. Guaco

9.   Rhubarb Root

10.   Yellow Dock

11.   Sarsaparilla Root

12.   Irish Sea Moss

How to Cleanse Using the Cleansing Herbs Above for Any Form of ED?

To detoxify your body system for any form of ED, using the above herbs, you will need to know the following things:

1. Knowing the right combination

2. You will need to know how to prepare, mix and administer the herbal teas using the above cleansing herbs

3. How to administer or consume the herbs.

Knowing the Right Herb Combinations

All the cleansing herbs for ED are powerful individually and can produce excellent results, but Dr. Sebi recommends that we do the right combination to enhance their detoxifying effects. In grouping them, I recommend grouping them based on their purposes:

1. The best herbs for cleansing people suffering from any form of ED are Burdock Root, Cascara Sagrada bark, Yellow Dock Root, Rhubarb Root, Dandelion Root, and Leaves.

2. Like many doctors will advise you to cleanse the colon, Dr. Sebi recommends cleansing every cell that makes up the organs and the systems that form the biological being (intracellular cleaning). Now, aside from cleaning the entire body system, Dr. Sebi recommends boosting the immune system to fight against any form of ED in you. That is why Elderberries, Mullein leaves, Eucalyptus leaves, and Guaco leaves are parts of

the cleansing herbs for ED.

3. Mineral boosting purpose: According to Dr. Sebi, ED is caused by accumulated mucous in the male reproductive system, and, to cleanse the body properly, there is a need to replenish some of the minerals that the cleansing herbs will flush out of the system. Thus, the need for Irish Sea Moss gel and Sarsaparilla Root.

How to Prepare and Administer the Cleansing Herbs for ED?

To prepare the herbal teas, you will need the following ingredients:

1. 2 tbsp dried Burdock Root

2. 1 tbsp Cascara Sagrada bark

3. 1 tbsp Chaparral leaves and stem

4. 1 tbsp Dandelion root, leaves, or flowers (mix if desired)

5. 2 tbsp elderberries (dry or fresh)

6. 1 tbsp Mullein leaves and flowers

7. 1 tbsp Eucalyptus leaves

8. 1 tbsp Guaco leaves

9. 1 tbsp Rhubarb Root

10.   1 tbsp Yellow Dock root

11.   1 tbsp Sarsaparilla Root

12.   2 tbsp Irish Sea Moss gel

The instructions are:

1. Get 3-4 cups of water or 24-32 ounces of water, and boil the water in a clean pot.

2. Simmer all the herbal roots and barks (tougher to less tough): Burdock Root, Cascara Sagrada, Rhubarb Root, Sarsaparilla Root, and Yellow Dock root to boiling water and reduce the heat

and allow the mixture to simmer for at least 25 minutes.

3. Add the softer herbs: Dandelion flowers/leaves, Chaparral, Elderberries, Mullein leaves/flowers, Eucalyptus, and Guaco and allow the mixture to simmer for an additional 10-15 minutes.

4. Get a strainer or fine mesh or cheesecloth and strain the liquid into a large jar or cup to remove the plant material.

5. Measure 2 tbsp of Irish Sea Moss gel and add it to the warm strained herbal tea to infuse its nutrients. Stir well until it is fully dissolved. Note that you can use the same ratio to do a larger quantity.

Administering the tea

To consume these herbal teas, drink 1 to 2 cups of the tea 2-3 times per day, depending on the strength of the cleanse and your body's tolerance level. If this is the first time you want to do a detox, you can start with 1 cup daily and increase gradually.

The best time to take your herbal teas is in the morning and before going to bed on an empty stomach to maximize the detoxification effects. For more intense cleansing, you can sip it throughout the day.

Please note that you can store any leftover tea in your refrigerator for a maximum period of 3 days and whenever you want to consume it, reheat the tea gently, without bringing it to a boil, to preserve its nutrients and effectiveness. Please don't microwave your chilled or frozen herbal teas as it will kill all the nutrients.

The Revitalizing Herbs for Erectile Dysfunction (ED), Low Sperm Count, Weak Erection, Etc.

The revitalizing herbs for erectile dysfunction (ED) such as: low sperm count, weak erections, premature ejaculation, poor sexual performance, low libido, low energy, and stamina level, etc. are:

1. Capadulla

2. Locust Bark

3. Yohimbi

4. Sarsaparilla Root

5. Irish Sea Moss

6. Pygeum

How to Revitalize the Body System Using the Revitalizing Herbs Above for Any Form of ED?

To revitalize the body system means to nourish and replenish all the nutrients and minerals that the body must have lost due to the cleansing process. Using the above herbs, you will need to know the following things.

1. You will need to know how to prepare, and mix,

the herbal teas using the above revitalizing herbs

2. How to administer or consume the herbs.

How to Prepare and Administer the Revitalizing Herbs After Cleansing for ED

As stated earlier, immediately after you finish your cleansing, you should go ahead and start taking the revitalizing herbs.

To prepare the revitalizing herbs, you will need the following ingredients:

1. 1 tbsp Capadulla bark

2. 1 tbsp Locust bark

3. 1 tbsp Yohimbe bark

4. 1 tbsp Sarsaparilla root

5. 1 tbsp Pygeum bark

6. 2 tbsp Irish Sea Moss gel

The instructions are:

1. Get a pot and pour 3-4 cups of water or 24 to 32 ounces of water and boil the water.

2. Add the revitalizing herbs; Capadulla bark, Locust bark, Yohimbe bark, Sarsaparilla root, and Pygeum bark to the boiling water in the pot and l lower the heat and allow the mixture to simmer for at least 35 minutes.

3. Turn off the heat and bring the pot with the mixture down.

4. Get a strainer or fine mesh or cheesecloth and strain the liquid (herbal tea) into a large jar or cup to remove the herbal residual.

5. Measure 2 tbsp of Irish Sea Moss gel and add it to the warm strained herbal tea to infuse its nutrients. Stir well until it is fully dissolved.

6. Allow the tea to get cool slightly to a comfortable drinking temperature before consumption

Administering the Tea

To consume these herbal teas, drink 1 to 2 cups of tea 2-3 times per day. If you are doing the 2 steps of healing for the first time, I strongly recommend you start taking smaller dosages. That is, 2 cups maximum per day because of sensitive herbs like Yohimbe, and gradually increase the dosage as your body adapts to it.

The best time to take your herbal teas is in the morning and before going to bed on an empty stomach to boost energy, vitality, and overall wellness throughout the day. Alternatively, a cup in the afternoon can also support prolonged energy and stamina.

CHAPTER FIVE

Herbal Remedy for Genital Herpes

The Cleansing Herbs for Genital Herpes

The cleansing herbs for genital herpes are:

1.   Sarsaparilla Root

2.   Burdock Root

3.   Dandelion

4.   Elderberry

5.   Mullein

6.   Chaparral

7.   Eucalyptus

8.   Guaco

9.   Cilantro

How to Cleanse Using the Cleansing Herbs Above for Genital Herpes

To cleanse using the above herbs for genital herpes,

you will need to know the following thing.

1. Knowing the right herbs combination

2. You will need to know how to prepare, and mix, the herbal teas using the above cleansing herbs

3. How to administer or consume the herbs.

Knowing the Right Herbs Combination

All the herbs are powerful even when used alone but to get an excellent result, late Dr. Sebi, recommend that we combine the herbs to create a powerful detoxifying and immune-boosting tea, rich in antioxidants, anti-inflammatory compounds, and essential nutrients.

1. Detoxification or Cleansing purpose: The best herbs for cleansing or detoxification for Genital herpes are Sarsaparilla, burdock root, Dandelion, and Chaparral which are known because of their potency to purify the blood, eliminate toxins and supports liver and kidney functionalities. In

addition, Dandelion is a natural diuretic, detox the liver, kidneys, and digestive system, Chaparral is an effective antioxidant and detoxifier that eliminate free radicals.

2. Immune Support and Anti-inflammatory Purpose: As cleansing is going on, it is recommended that the immune is boosted to fight against all possible symptoms of cleansing. Such herbs include: Elderberry (Fresh or Dried) and mullein that are rich in antioxidants and vitamin C, which in turn will boosts the immune system and fights off colds, flu, reduce inflammation, and support lung health by clearing out mucus. In addition, Eucalyptus Leaves serves as an antimicrobial agent.

3. Respiratory Support Purpose: Mullein, Eucalyptus, and Guaco helps to promotes lung health and helps clear respiratory congestion,

and reduces inflammation.

How to Prepare And Administer The Cleansing Herbs for Genital Herpes?

To preparing the herbal teas for the cleansing of the body system for genital herpes, you will need the following ingredients:

1. 1 tbsp Sarsaparilla Root

2. 1 tbsp Burdock Root

3. 1 tbsp Dandelion Root (can also use leaves and flowers)

4. 2 tbsp Elderberries (fresh or dried)

5. 1 tbsp Mullein leaves and flowers

6. 1 tbsp Chaparral leaves and stem

7. 1 tbsp Eucalyptus leaves

8. 1 tbsp Guaco leaves

9. 1 tbsp fresh cilantro leaves and stem

The Instructions are:

1. Get 3-4 cups of water or 24-32 ounce of water, boil the water in a clean pot. Use spring water which is preferable but if you can't, normal water can still work

2. Simmer all the herbal roots, barks and berries (tougher to less tough) Sarsaparilla Root, Burdock Root, and Elderberries to the boiling water and reduce the heat and allow the mixture to simmer for at least 30 minutes.

3. Add the leaves and flowering herbs (Dandelion leaves and flowers, Mullein leaves and flowers, Chaparral, Eucalyptus, Guaco, and cilantro leaves/stems) to the pot. Let the mixture simmer for an additional 10-15 minutes.

4. Use a strainer or cheesecloth to strain the tea into a cup or jar to remove the plant material.

Administering the Tea

To consume this herbal teas, drink 1 to 2 cups of tea 2-3 times per day. If you are doing the 2 steps of healing for the first time, I strongly recommend you start taking smaller dosage. Start with 2 cup per day before you can gradually increase it to 3 or more cups if needed.

The best time to take your herbal teas are in the morning and before going to bed on an empty stomach for detoxification or throughout the day for immune and energy booster.

Please note that if the tea is too strong or bitter, you can decide to add a natural sweetener such as: maple or agave syrup or a squeeze of lime juice to balance the flavor.

The Revitalizing Herbs for Genital Herpes

The revitalizing herbs for herpes are:

1.   Pao Pereira

2.   Pau d'Arco

3.   Holy Basil

4.   Oregano Essential Oil

5.   Ginger Essential Oil

6.   Sea Salt Bath

7.   Irsih Sea moss

How to Revitalize the Body System Using the Revitalizing Herbs Above for Genital Herpes?

Unlike all the other revitalizing process, for the skin and genital herpes, there are some few different steps that are not same with other type of diseases.

The best approach is to use a combination of internal herbal teas to destroy the virus internally, and topical treatments, to eliminate the virus externally and detoxifying baths. All the herbs for the revitalization and essential oils brings antiviral, immune-boosting, and soothing properties to help manage and alleviate genital herpes symptoms.

What Are the Internal Herbal Teas?

The internal herbal teas are the revitalizing teas that you are made to consume immediately after you finish cleansing for genital herpes to boost your immune as well as provide antiviral action support. To prepare these teas, you will need the following ingredients handy:

1. 1 tbsp Pao Pereira bark

2. 1 tbsp Pau d'Arco bark

3. 1 tbsp Holy Basil leaves (Tulsi)

4. 1 tbsp Guaco leaves

5. 1 tbsp Cilantro leaves and stems

6. 2 tbsp Irish Sea Moss

The Instructions are:

1. Get a clean pot and pour 3-4cups of water or 24-32ounce of water, boil the water

2. Once the water is boiling, simmer the barks (Pao Pereira and Pau d'Arco barks) to the boiling water and reduce the heat and allow it to simmer for minimum of 30 minutes.

3. Add the softer herbs such as: Holy Basil, Guaco, and Cilantro leaves/stems and allow the mixture simmer for an additional 10-15 minutes before dropping the pot down

4. Get a strainer or cheesecloth to strain the tea into a cup or jar to remove the plant material.

5. Add the 2tbsp of Irish sea moss gel and stir it properly before consuming it.

Administering the Tea

To consume this herbal teas, drink 1 to 2 cups of tea 2-3 times per day especially during outbreak as it helps to boost the immune system and reduce viral activities. If you are doing the 2 steps of healing for the first time, I strongly recommend you start taking smaller dosage. Start with 2 cup per day before you can gradually increase it to 3 or more cups if needed.

The best time to take your herbal teas are in the morning and before going to bed on an empty stomach for detoxification or throughout the day for immune and energy booster.

Please note that if the tea is too strong or bitter, you can decide to add a natural sweetener such as: maple or agave syrup or a squeeze of lime juice to balance the flavor.

Tropical Revitalization for Genital Herpes

The first tropical treatment is the "Essential Oil Application" design to treat all form of virus, irritation and inflammation.

The ingredients are:

1. 2 drops of oregano essential oil

2. 2 drops of ginger essential oil

3. 1 tbsp carrier oil (coconut oil)

The instructions are:

1. Get a small bowl or bottle, to dilute all the essential oil by mixing the 2 drops each of both the oregano and ginger essential oil together with 1 tablespoon of coconut oil.

2. Gently apply the diluted mixture (oregano, ginger essential oil and coconut oil) to the affected area 2-3 times per day during outbreaks to help soothe the skin and fight the virus topically. Please note that care has to be taken when apply any tropical treatment to prevent any form of excessive irritation, especially with the potent Oregano Oil.

Sea Salt Bath (for soothing and detoxifying)
The ingredients are:

1. 2 cups of sea salt

2. First optional: drop a few drops of ginger or oregano essential oil because o of it antiviral potency

The instructions are:

1. Fill your bathtub with hot water that you can bath in and dissolve the 2 cups of sea salt into the water.

2. Add 2-3 drops of ginger or oregano essential oil or both to the bathtub.

3. Mix the essential oil thoroughly to ensure the oils are properly dispersed into the water before getting in.

4. Soak yourself into the bathtub for at least 30 minutes so that the sea salt will draw out toxins

and soothe irritation, while the essential oils provide antiviral benefits.

Please note that: consistency is the key when it comes to managing genital herpes and it is also, very important to maintain a healthy lifestyle, mange stress, and boost your immune system during the revitalizing process by consuming Irish sea moss.

Take extra caution by diluting the oregano essential oil properly before using it because of it strong potency. Once you notice excessive burning or irritation, please stop using this essential oil or reduce the amount use immediately.

CHAPTER SIX
Herbal Remedy for High Blood Pressure (Hypertension)
The Cleansing Herbs for High Blood Pressure (Hypertension)

The cleansing herbs for high blood pressure (hypertension) are:

1. Cascara Sagrada

2. Rhubarb Root

3. Prodigiosa

4. Burdock Root

5. Chaparral

6. Dandelion

7. Elderberry

8. Guaco

9. Eucalyptus

10. Mullein

How to Cleanse Using the Cleansing Herbs Above to Reverse High Blood Pressure

Naturally, all these herbs are potent (contain detoxifying, diuretic, and anti-inflammatory properties that help to regulate blood pressure, boost cardiovascular health, and cleanse the entire body system) on their own, but it is more potent to mix these herbs to get the desired result.

Before cleansing, there are basics that you need to know:

1. Knowing the right herbs combination

2. How to prepare and administer the herbs?

3. How to store and reheat the tea, etc.

Knowing The Right Herbs Combination

1. Laxative and cleansing purpose: Herbs such as Cascara Sagrada, Rhubarb root, and Burdock root have mild laxative, and help to purify the

blood, detox the body system, and support bowel's health, digestion, liver, and kidney functionalities.

2. Herds such as Prodigious leaves/stem, Chaparral leaves/stem, and dandelion flower/leaves and the entire dandelion plant have antioxidants and diuretics and also help to regulate blood sugar and blood pressure, support cardiovascular health, liver, and remove excess fluids from the body, which can lower blood pressure.

3. Anti-inflammation, Support immune and circulation: Herbs like Elderberries, Guaco leaves, eucalyptus leaves, and mullein leaves are high in antioxidants and anti-inflammation, supporting the immune system, circulation, lung health as well as cardiovascular functionalities and reducing stress.

How to Prepare and Administer the Cleansing Herbs for High Blood Pressure (Hypertension)

To prepare the herbal tea to cleanse for high blood pressure, you will need the following ingredients:

1. Tbsp Cascara Sagrada bark

2. 1 Tbsp Rhubarb Root

3. 1 tbsp. Burdock Root

4. 1 tbsp. Chaparral leaves and stem

5. 1 tbsp. Prodigious leaves and stem

6. 1 Tbsp Dandelion flowers, root, and leaves

7. 2 tbsp. Elderberries (fresh or dried)

8. 1 Tbsp Guano leaves

9. 1 tbsp. Mullein leaves and flowers

10.   1 Tbsp of Eucalyptus leaves

The instructions are:

1. Get a clean pot and pour in 4-5 cups of water or 32- 40 ounces of water and boil it.

2. Add all the tough herbs; Cascara Sagrada, Rhubarb Root, Burdock Root, and Chaparral to the boiling water and reduce the heat for the herbs to simmer for at least 35 minutes.

3. Add all the soft herbs: Prodigiosa, Dandelion, Elderberries, Guano, Mullein, and Eucalyptus leaves, stir, and allow it to simmer for at least 15 minutes.

4. Remove the pot from the heat and get a strainer or fine mesh/cheesecloth to strain the mixture into a cup or jar to remove the plant materials.

Administering the Tea

To consume these herbal teas, drink 1 to 2 cups of tea 2-3 times per day. If you are doing the 2 steps of healing for the first time, I strongly recommend you start taking a smaller dosage. Start with 2 cups per day before you can gradually increase it to 3 or more cups per day if need be, as the cleansing herbs will serve as a gentle detoxifier, reducing blood pressure by eliminating excess toxins and fluids from the body.

The best time to take your herbal teas is in the morning and before going to bed on an empty stomach for detoxification or throughout the day for immune and energy boosters.

But for high blood pressure cleansing, the best time to consume these teas is in the morning and afternoon. At all costs, avoid consuming these herbs late in the night as they can disrupt your sleep.

Please note that if the tea is too strong or bitter, you can decide to add a natural sweetener such as maple or agave syrup or a squeeze of lime juice to balance the flavor.

Usually, you can store unused herbal teas in the

refrigerator for a maximum period of 3 days.

Do not microwave herbal teas as all you need to do is to warm it gently before drinking it. Please just warm not boiled

The Revitalizing Herbs for High Blood Pressure (Hypertension)

The revitalizing herbs for High Blood Pressure (Hypertension) are:

1. Flor de Manita

2. Lily of the Valley

3. Hierba Del Sapo

4. Shepherd's Purse

5. For de Tila

6. Sarsaparilla Root

7. Valerian Root

8. Yarrow

9. Lupus

How to Revitalize the Body System Using the Herbs Above After Cleansing for High Blood Pressure?

Revitalizing the body system after a cleanse for high blood pressure is very important to balance cardiovascular support with nervous system relaxation, calm the mind, and soothe the heart while reasonably rejuvenating the body system back to its original alkaline state where high blood pressure cannot survive, and restore vitality after detoxification.

Before the revitalization process, it will be very important to know. There are basics that you need to know:

1. Knowing the Right Herbs Combination

2. How to prepare and administer the herbs

3. The storage, and reheating etc.

Knowing the Right Herbs Combination

1. Heart strengthened and promotion of circulation and regulate the heartbeat: Herbs like Flor De Manita, Lily of the Valley, Shepherd's Purse, and Yarrow help to strengthen and support circulation, and cardiovascular system, boost heart health, regulate heart functionalities, heartbeat, and lower blood pressure. Additionally, yarrow has anti-inflammatory properties that help with recovery after cleansing.

2. Reduced cholesterol and replenish the body, with the lost minerals during cleansing: Herbs like Hierba Del Sapo, and Sarsaparilla root, help to support liver and heart function, reduce cholesterol, purify the blood, and revitalize the body, and support energy after detox, which is essential for long-term recovery after cleansing.

3. Diuretic and stress management and restful

sleep: Herbs like; Flor De Tila, Valerian root and lupus have nerving that helps to calm the mind, and nervous system, and reduces stress and anxiety which in return can promote restful sleep which is crucial for the body's recovery after detox.

How to Prepare and Administer the Revitalizing Herbs After Cleansing for High Blood Pressure

To prepare and administer the herbal after cleansing for high blood pressure, you will need the following ingredients:

1. 1 Tbsp of Sarsaparilla Root

2. 1 Tbsp of Valerian Root

3. 1 Tbsp Flor De Manita flowers

4. 1 Tbsp Lily of the Valley flowers

5. 1 Tbsp Hierba Del Sapo leaves/stems

6. 1 Tbsp Shepherd's Purse stems, leaves, flowers, and seed pods

7. 1 tbsp. Flor de Tila flowers

8. 1 tbsp. Yarrow leaves and flowers

9. 1 tbsp. Lupus (Hops) flowers

The instructions are:

1. Get a clean pot and pour in 4-5 cups of water or 32- 40 ounces of water and boil it.

2. Add all the tough herbs; Sarsaparilla Root and Valerian Root to the boiling water and reduce the heat and allow it to simmer for at least 30 minutes.

3. Add all the soft herbs: Flor De Manita, Lily of the Valley, Hierba Del Sapo, Shepherd's Purse, Flor De Tila, Yarrow, and Lupus flowers, and simmer the mixture for at least 15 minutes.

4. Drop it from the heat and use a fine mesh strainer or cheesecloth to strain the tea into a cup or jar to remove the plant materials.

Administering the Tea

To consume these herbal teas, drink 1 to 2 cups of tea 2-3 times per day. If you are doing the 2 steps of healing for the first time, I strongly recommend you start taking a smaller dosage. Start with 2 cups per day before you can gradually increase it to 3 or more cups if needed.

The best time to take your herbal teas is in the morning, which will help to support blood flow and energy, and before going to bed on an empty stomach as it will help the body to relax and recover, especially aiding in restful sleep.

Please note that if the tea is too strong or bitter, you can decide to add a natural sweetener such as maple or agave syrup or a squeeze of lime juice to balance the flavor.

You can store the remaining tea in your refrigerator for a maximum period of 3 days and when you want to consume the stored herbal tea, warm it gently, don't boil it, and do not use a microwave to preserve the active compounds.

CHAPTER SEVEN
Natural Remedy for Diabetes and Dialysis
The Cleansing Herbs for Diabetes and Dialysis

The cleansing herbs for diabetes and dialysis are:

1. Cascara Sagrada

2. Rhubarb root

3. Burdock root

4. Blessed Thistle

5. Dandelion

6. Elderberry

7. Mullein

8. Chaparral

9. Guaco

How to Cleanse Using the Cleansing Herbs Above to Treat Diabetes and Dialysis

To cleanse for diabetes and dialysis, there are some key factors which include:

1. Knowing the right herbs combination

2. How to prepare and administer the herbs

3. Storage of unused herbal teas and reheating, etc.

Knowing the Right Herbs Combination

All the herbs are very potent in their unique ways, but the late Dr. Sebi recommends the right combination to help eliminate the root cause of diabetes and dialysis. These herbs are combined based on purpose:

1. Herbs like Cascara Sagrada, Rhubarb root, and burdock roots are natural laxatives that help stimulate bowel movements, detoxify the liver, kidney, and blood, and also help to improve digestive function, which is key for dialysis patients.

2. Herbs like thistle and dandelion help detoxify the liver and kidney, enhance digestion, and regulate blood sugar, which is beneficial for people suffering from diabetes.

3. Antioxidants and immune system booster herbs such as Elderberries and chaparral are packed with antioxidants that aid in supporting the immune system and detoxifying the liver and the body system in general by eliminating toxins.

4. Detox respiratory system and anti-inflammation: herbs like Mullein and Guaco is known for its potency to reduce inflammation, and cleansing of the respiratory system's health, and promote detoxification through the lungs.

How to Prepare and Administer the Cleansing Herbs for Diabetes and Dialysis?

To prepare and administer the cleansing herbs for diabetes and dialysis, you will need the following ingredients:

1. 1 tbsp Cascara Sagrada bark

2. 1 tbsp Rhubarb root

3. 1 tbsp Burdock root

4. 1 tbsp Blessed Thistle leaves/stems/flowers

5. 1 tbsp Dandelion flowers/root/

6. 1 tbsp fresh or dried

7. 1 tbsp Mullein leaves/flowers

8. 1 tbsp Chaparral leaves/stem

9. 1 tbsp Guaco leaves

The instructions are:

Get a clean pot and pour in 4-5 cups of water or 32-40ounces of water and boil it.

2.   Add all the tough herbs; Cascara Sagrada bark, Rhubarb root, and Burdock root to the boiling water and reduce the heat before you simmer it for at least

30 minutes.

3. Add the Blessed Thistle, Dandelion, Elderberries, Mullein, Chaparral, and Guaco and allow the mixture to simmer for at least 15 minutes before turning off the heat

4. Get a fine mesh, strainer, or cheesecloth and strain the herbal tea into a cup or jar to remove all plant material.

Administering the Tea

Drink 2-3 cups of herbal tea, 2-3 times daily, depending on your capacity. However, if you are new to herbs or have never done cleansing before, I recommend starting with at least two cups per day before you can decide to increase it as your body system gets used to the herbal teas. Please note that this herbal tea combination will help to cleanse and detox the liver, kidneys, and digestive system, which is very important for individuals with diabetes and undergoing dialysis.

The best times to consume these herbal teas are on an empty stomach, preferably in the morning to stimulate cleansing, and in the evening before bed to continue with the cleansing process throughout the night.

Just like the other teas, you can store them in the refrigerator and warm them gently. No microwave.

The Revitalizing Herbs for Diabetes

The revitalizing herbs for diabetes are:

1. Nopal/Prickly Pear Cactus

2. Huereque/Wereke

3. Prodigiosa

4. The Sensitive Plant/Ti Marie

5. Stinging Nettle

6. Anamu/Guinea Hen Weed

7.   Hierba Del Sapo

How to Revitalize the Body System after Cleansing for Diabetes?

To revitalize the body system after cleansing for diabetes, you will need to know and follow the steps below:

1. Knowing the right herbal combination.

2. How to prepare and administer the herbal teas

3. How to store unused herbal teas and reheat them before consumption, etc.

knowing the Right Herbal Combination

1. Cleansing of the blood and overall body detoxification purpose: herbs such as; Huereque/Wereke root help to purify the blood and the entire body system.

2. Support liver and kidney functions and regulation of blood sugar level: hers such as; Nopal/Prickly Pear cactus, Huereque/Wereke

root, Hierba del sapo and Prodigiosa leaves are potent herbs that stimulate pancreatic functions, support both heart, kidney, and liver function, and regulate blood sugar levels and wereke helps to restore balance in the body and lastly, stinging nettle promotes overall vitality and restores nutrients in the body with its rich iron and minerals properties.

3. Anti-inflammation and immune and nervous system booster: Herbs such as The Sensitive Plant/Ti Marie, An amu/Guinea Hen Weed help to reduce inflammation, calm the nervous system, boost the immune system, and provide energy to revitalize the body, which is important for post-cleansing recovery.

How to Prepare and Administer the Revitalizing Herbs for Diabetes

To prepare and administer the revitalizing herbs after cleansing for diabetes, you will need the following ingredients:

1. 1 tbsp Huereque/Wereke root

2. 1 tbsp Nopal/Prickly Pear Cactus (dried or fresh)

3. 1 tbsp Prodigiosa leaves/stems

4. 1 tbsp The Sensitive Plant/Ti Marie leaves

5. 1 tbsp Stinging Nettle leaves

6. 1 tbsp Anamu/Guinea Hen Weed leaves/stem

7. 1 tbsp Hierba Del Sapo leaves/stems

The instructions are:

1. Get a clean pot and pour in 4-5 cups of water or 32-40 ounces of water and boil it.

2. Add Huereque/Wereke root to the boiling water, reduce the heat and allow it to simmer for at least 30 minutes.

3. Add all the soft herbs: Nopal/Prickly Pear, Prodigiosa, The Sensitive Plant/Ti Marie, Stinging Nettle, Anamu, and Hierba Del Sapo, and allow it to simmer for at least another 15 minutes.

4. Get a fine mesh or strainer or cheesecloth to strain the tea into a cup or jar to remove the plant material.

The Administration is:

Drink 2-3 cups of the herbal tea, 2-3 times daily, depending on your capacity. However, if you are new to herbs or have never done cleansing before, I recommend starting with at least two cups per day before you can decide to increase it as your body system gets used to the herbal teas. Please note that this herbal tea combination will help your body to recover and regulate blood sugar levels while restoring energy and overall vitality.

The best times to drink these herbal teas are in the morning on an empty stomach to support energy and blood sugar balance throughout the day, and in the evening to promote continued replenishing of the body system.

Just like the other herbal teas, store unused teas in a refrigerator and do not use the microwave to warm them whenever you want to consume it, just warm it gently and do not allow it to boil.

As the process is going on, always monitor your blood sugar level. It is important to regularly monitor your blood sugar levels as these herbs can have a strong effect on blood sugar regulation.

Revitalizing Herbs for People On Dialysis Machine

According to Dr. Sebi, people suffering from dialysis need their blood to be purified and need lots of energy (liquid iron and potassium phosphate).

However, the herbs to revitalize the body system for people on a dialysis machine after cleansing from diabetes and dialysis are:

1. Lily of the Valley

2. Sarsaparilla

3. Conconsa/Cancansa

4. Irish Sea Moss

5. Bladderwrack

6. Dandelion

7. Stinging nettle

How to Revitalize the Body System for Dialysis after Cleansing for Diabetes and Dialysis?

To revitalize the body system after cleansing for diabetes and dialysis, you need to know the following points:

1. Knowing the right herbal combination

2. How to prepare and administer the herbal teas

3. The storage, reheating, etc.

Knowing the Right Herbal Combination

1. Support and revitalize the heart, liver, and kidneys and purify the blood purpose: Herbs like sarsaparilla root, conconsa/cancansa, lily of the valley, and dandelion are potent with nutrients to support and revitalize the liver, kidney, and thyroid and purify the blood.

2. Revitalize and replenish the body and boost the immune system: Herbs like Irish Sea moss, sarsaparilla root, stinging nettle, and Bladderwrack are rich in minerals and nutrients that help the body to recover from all the energy, minerals, and nutrients it has lost during the cleansing process.

How to Prepare and Administer Herbal Teas for Dialysis?

To prepare and administer herbal teas for dialysis, you will need the following ingredients:

1. 1 tbsp Sarsaparilla root

2. 1 tbsp Conconsa/Cancansa bark/root

3. 1 tbsp Irish Sea Moss gel

4. 1 tbsp Bladderwrack fronds/leaves

5. 1 tbsp Dandelion flowers/root/leaves

6. 1 tbsp Stinging Nettle leaves

7. 1 tbsp Lily of the Valley flowers

The instructions are:

1. Get a clean pot and pour in 4-5 cups of water or 32-40 ounces of water and boil it.

2. Add all the tough herbs: Sarsaparilla root and Conconsa/Cancansa bark/root to the boiling

water, reduce the heat, and allow it to simmer for at least 25 minutes.

3. Add all the soft herbs: Dandelion flowers/root/leaves, Stinging Nettle leaves, Bladderwrack, and Lily of the Valley flowers, and allow the mixture to simmer for an additional 15 minutes before turning off the heat

4. Get a strainer or fine mesh or cheesecloth to strain the herbal teas into a cup or jar and remove the wood.

5. Add the Irish Sea Moss gel and stir properly before consumption.

6. You might still want to strain it, but it is not too important.

Administering the Tea

Drink 2-3 cups of this herbal tea twice or thrice per day. It is important to start with smaller amounts and increase the dose gradually if you have never done the 2 steps of the healing methodology (cleansing and revitalizing), especially for individuals on dialysis or managing diabetes. This tea is rich in minerals and supports the kidneys, so monitor how your body responds as you consume the tea.

The best time to consume this herbal tea is in the morning on an empty stomach to help boost energy and support the kidneys and liver after detox, and in the evening, to help the body continue the revitalization process overnight.

The storage and warming of the teas is still the same method

Please make sure you always monitor the symptoms because of the strong medicinal effects of these herbs, especially for people on dialysis and with diabetes.

CHAPTER EIGHT
Natural Remedy for Autoimmune Disease
The Cleansing Herbs for Autoimmune Disease

Before going for cleansing and revitalizing of the general body system to get rid of the root cause of autoimmune disease, it is very important to take note of these few important notes:

1. Eat only alkaline diets (Food approved by Dr. Sebi) as a switch can lead to body relapse and the disease returned.

2. If there is any foreign object (medical device) planted in your body, you will need to remove it immediately.

3. Avoid any trigger foods (including alkaline diets that can trigger autoimmune diseases)

4. Undergo the cleansing process at least twice in a

year or any time that you feel you are having an inflammatory response, you should observe at least, 3 days fast.

The cleansing herbs for autoimmune diseases are:

1. Cascara Sagrada

2. Rhubarb root

3. Prodigiosa

4. Burdock root

5. Chaparral

6. Dandelion

7. Elderberry

8. Guaco

9. Eucalyptus

10.   Mullein

How to Cleanse Using the Cleansing Herbs Above to Treat All Forms of Autoimmune Disease

To do a detox to eradicate or treat and prevent any form of autoimmune disease, you will need to know that the focus should be on consuming herbs that have the potency to detoxify/cleanse the liver, reduce inflammation, and boost the immune system. To do this you need to know the following:

1. Knowing the right herbal combination

2. How to prepare and administer the cleansing herbal teas

3. How to store and warm the herbal teas

Knowing the Right Herbal Combination

1. Detox/cleanse liver, kidney, digestive system, and pancreatic health: herbs such as; Rhubarb root, Prodigiosa leaves, and dandelions plant help to detoxify the liver, kidney, support digestive and pancreatic health, which is very

important in managing autoimmune diseases.

2. Support the colon's health and stimulate the movement of the bowel to cleanse the entire body system: herbs like cascara Sagrada bark has active nutrients that help to detox the colon and the general body system.

3. Anti-inflammatory, antioxidant and immune booster: herbs such as Burdock root, chaparral, and elderberries have anti-inflammatory and antioxidant properties that can cleanse the body of free radicals, reduce inflammation and also elderberries helps to boost the immune system and burdock root purifies the blood which are all very important and in treating any form of autoimmune diseases.

4. Support respiratory system, rich in antimicrobial and soothing properties: Herbs such as Guaco leaves, eucalyptus leaves and mullein are very

rich in antimicrobial and soothing properties that help to support the respiratory system which is also important when it comes to autoimmune diseases.

How to Prepare and Administer the Herbal Tea for Autoimmune Diseases

To prepare and administer the cleansing herbs for autoimmune disease, you will need the following ingredients:

1. 1 tbsp Cascara Sagrada bark

2. 1 tbsp Rhubarb root

3. 1 tbsp Prodigiosa leaves and stems

4. 1 tbsp Burdock root

5. 1 tbsp Chaparral leaves and stems

6. 1 tbsp Dandelion flowers, root, and leaves

7. 1 tbsp Elderberries

8. 1 tbsp Guaco leaves

9. 1 tbsp Eucalyptus leaves

10. 1 tbsp Mullein leaves/flowers

The instructions are:

1. Get a clean port and measure 4-6 cups of water or 48 ounces of water and boil it.

2. Add all the hard hers such as; rhubarb root, cascara sagrada bark, and burdock root to the boiling water, lower the heat, and allow the mixture to simmer for at least 30 minutes.

3. Add all the soft herbs; dandelion, prodigiosa, chaparral, Guaco, elderberries, mullein, and eucalyptus leaves to the mixture and allow it to simmer for an additional 10 minutes.

4. Turn off the heat, get a strainer, fine mesh, or cheesecloth to strain the tea into a cup or jar to remove all the plant material.

Administering the Tea

Drink 1 cup twice or thrice per day. Make sure you monitored the autoimmune diseases as autoimmune diseases are very sensitive to changes in the body. I strongly recommend that you monitor your symptoms carefully as you introduce the cleansing herbal teas and adjust as necessary as possible.

As you continue to consume the herbs, your body system including the liver and kidney will be completely detoxed while your immune system boosted.

The best time to consume this herbal tea is in the morning to support your daily detoxification and in the evening before going to bed to continue the cleansing process while the body rests.

The storage and warming of the teas is still the same

method.

The Revitalizing Herbs for Autoimmune Diseases

The revitalizing herbs for autoimmune diseases are:

1. Contribo (Duck flower vine)

2. Cordoncillo Negro

3. Pavana

4. Kalawalla

How to Use the Herbs Above to Revitalize the Body System After Cleansing for Autoimmune Diseases?

To revitalize the body system after cleansing for autoimmune diseases, it is of great importance for you to focus on boosting your immune system, and energy level replenishing all the essential nutrients that you might have lost due to the disease or cleansing process. First, you will need to:

1. Understand the revitalizing herbs

2. How to prepare and administer the herbs

3. The best time to consume the herbs, its storage, and how it can be warmed.

Understand the revitalizing herbs

1. Contribo (Duck flower vine): this herb is very effective for the cleansing of the residual toxins from the body after cleansing for autoimmune disease. Because of how powerful the effect of these herbs in revitalizing the body after cleansing for autoimmune diseases. I strongly recommend caution while using this herb.

2. Cordoncillo Negro leaves: this is another effective herb for revitalizing the body system after cleansing for autoimmune diseases because of its anti-inflammatory and antimicrobial properties and its potency to boost the energy level, immune and respiratory systems, which are key for people recovering from any form of

autoimmune diseases.

3. Pavana leaves/root: You can use either the root or the leaf or mix both, as they all have regenerative properties that speed healing and revitalize energy and overall healing and vitality.

4. Kalawalla rhizome: The rhizomes of kalawalla is an effective herb for revitalizing the body after cleansing for autoimmune diseases because of its potency to regulate, balance, and support the immune system, which is paramount for autoimmune diseases.

How to Prepare and Administer the Revitalizing Herbs After Cleansing for Autoimmune Disease?

To prepare and administer the revitalizing herbal teas, you will need the following ingredients:

1. 1 tbsp Contribo (Duck flower vine)

2. 1 tbsp Cordoncillo Negro leaves

3. 1 tbsp Pavana root/leaves

4. 1 tbsp Kalawalla rhizome

The instructions are:

1. Get a clean pot, measure 4-6 cups of water or 32-48 ounces of water, and boil it.

2. Add the Kalawalla rhizome to the boiling water, reduce the heat, and allow it to simmer for at least 30 minutes.

3. Add all the other herbs: pavana, cordoncillo negro, and contribo, and allow it to simmer for an additional 10 minutes.

4. Get a strainer, fine mesh, or cheesecloth to strain the herbal tea into a cup or jar to remove the herb's residual.

Administering the Tea

Drink 1 cup twice a day but start with 1 cup for the

first 3 days of your revitalization process. Make sure you monitor your body's reaction as you consume the herbs for the first 3 days because they are all four powerful herbs. However, if there are no negative effects, you can increase your consumption to 2 cups per day.

The best time to consume these herbal teas is in the morning on an empty stomach to support your body's energy and immune system throughout the day and the other cup before 4 pm as consuming the tea after 4 pm can lead to overstimulation.

You can store unused herbal teas in a refrigerator maximum period of 3 days. Anything after three days, do away with the unused herbal teas.

Make sure you warm or reheat the herbal tea that you store whenever you want to consume it using a stove or gas cooker over low heat to maintain the herbal properties.

Follow every other instruction as stated at the beginning of this chapter.

CHAPTER NINE
Herbal Remedy for Female Reproductive System Disorder
The Cleansing Herbs for Female Reproductive System Disorders

The cleansing herbs for female reproductive system disorders such as infertility, PCOS, fibroids, virginal discharge, endometriosis, etc. are:

1. Cascara Sagrada

2. Rhubarb root

3. Prodigiosa

4. Burdock root

5. Chaparral

6. Dandelion

7. Elderberry

8. Guaco

9. Eucalyptus

10.   Mullein

How to Cleanse Using the Cleansing Herbs Above to Treat All Forms of Female Reproductive System Disorder

To cleanse for the treatment of all forms of female reproductive system disorders, such as PCOS, fibroids, endometriosis, or other hormonal imbalances, you will need to know the following key things:

1. Understanding the cleansing herbal combination

2. How to prepare and administer the cleansing herbs

3. The storage, warming, and best time to consume the cleansing herbs

Understanding the Cleansing Herbal Combination

1. Digestion and blood purification: Herbs such as cascara sagrada, burdock root, and prodigiosa are very effective in cleansing the blood and the

digestive system and eradicating toxins in the female reproductive system, which are the key reasons Dr. Sebi included these herbs as part of the herbs to cleanse for female reproductive system, disorders.

2. Herbs such as Chaparral, burdock root, rhubarb root, and dandelion are very rich in antioxidant properties that help to cleanse and support liver and kidney functionalities and balance hormones, which are very important in female reproductive health.

3. Regulation of blood sugar, anti-inflammation, antimicrobial, and immune booster: Herbs such as elderberries are very effective in detoxification and boosting the immune system; eucalyptus, guaco and mullein have the potency to eliminate free radicals, reduce inflammation, and fight infection, which is also key in female

reproductive health.

How to Prepare and Administer the Cleansing Herbal Teas

To cleanse and administer the cleansing herbal teas for the female reproductive system disorders, you will need the following ingredients:

1. 1 tbsp Cascara Sagrada bark

2. 1 tbsp Rhubarb root

3. 1 tbsp Prodigiosa leaves

4. 1 tbsp Burdock root

5. 1 tbsp Chaparral leaves and stem

6. 1 tbsp Dandelion flowers/root/leaves

7. 1 tbsp Elderberries

8. 1 tbsp Guaco leaves

9. 1 tbsp Eucalyptus leaves

10.   1 tbsp Mullein leaves/flowers

The instructions are:

1. Get a clean pot, measure 4-6 cups of water or 32-48 ounces of water, and boil it.

2. Add all the hard herbs; cascara sagrada bark, rhubarb root, and burdock root to the boiling water, reduce the heat and allow it to simmer for at least 30 minutes.

3. Add all the soft herbs; prodigiosa leaves, chaparral leaves/stem, dandelion flowers/root/leaves, guaco leaves, eucalyptus leaves, mullein leaves/flowers, and elderberries, and allow it to simmer for an additional 10 minutes before bringing the pot down from the heat.

4. Get a strainer or fine mesh or cheesecloth and strain the tea into a cup or jar to remove herbal residual.

Administering the Tea

Drink 1 cup of the herbal cleansing tea twice per day, but you will have to monitor your system to see your tolerance level by drinking one cup per day, for the first 3 days of the cleanse before you can increase it to 2 cups per day.

The best times to consume this herbal tea are in the morning to stimulate the cleansing process and in the evenings before going to sleep to continue with the cleanse while you get a sound night's rest.

Just like the other herbal teas, storage and warming are the same thing. Don't forget to get enough rest during this cleansing exercise and drink lots of spring water (at least 1 gallon per day)

The Revitalizing Herbs for Female Reproductive System Disorder

The revitalizing herbs for female reproductive system disorders such as; infertility, PCOS, fibroids, virginal discharge, endometriosis etc. are:

1. Red clover

2. Pau D'Arco

3. Chaparral

4. Red Raspberry leaves

5. Shepherd's purse

6. Peony

7. Stinging Nettle

8. Irish Sea Moss

9. Sarsaparilla

How to Use the Revitalizing Herbs Above to Revitalize the Body System After Cleansing for Female Reproductive System Disorders?

To revitalize the body system after cleansing for female reproductive system disorders, it is of great importance for you to focus on supporting your female reproductive system, boosting your immune system, regulating your hormonal balance, and replenishing all the nutrients lost due to the disorder. First, you will need to:

1. Understand the revitalizing herbal combination

2. How to prepare and administer the herbs

3. The best time to consume the herbs, its storage, and how they can be warmed.

Understanding the Revitalizing Herbal Combination

1. Balancing of hormones, and immune boosters: Herbal teas made with herbs like red clover flowers, Pau D'Arco inner bark, sarsaparilla root, and chaparral leaves have very powerful properties that have the potency to balance hormones most especially estrogen, strengthen the immune system, reduce inflammation, and

support the female reproductive system which is very important when it comes to female reproductive health.

2. Support the female reproductive system and regulate menstrual cycles: Herbal teas made with herbs like; Red raspberry leaves, peony root, and shepherd's purse leaves have properties that can support the female reproductive system, regulate menstrual cycles, heavy menstrual bleeding, and menstrual irregularities, that is why all these herbs are important in revitalizing the body to treat female reproductive system disorders.

3. Essential nutrients and immune booster: Herbal teas made with stinging nettle, Irish Sea moss gel, and sarsaparilla root are very rich in over 100+ nutrients to support uterine health, tissue repairs, and cleanse the entire system that makes up the biological body, and boost overall reproductive

health. Lastly, the sarsaparilla root doubles up to purify the liver and blood.

How to Prepare and Administer the Revitalizing Herbs After Cleansing for Female Reproductive System Disorder

To prepare and administer the revitalizing herbs after cleansing for female reproductive system disorder, you will need the following ingredients:

1. 1 tbsp Pau D'Arco inner bark
2. 1 tbsp Peony root
3. 1 tbsp Sarsaparilla root
4. 1 tbsp Red clover flowers
5. 1 tbsp Chaparral leaves and stem
6. 1 tbsp Red Raspberry leaves
7. 1 tbsp Shepherd's purse (aerial parts)
8. 1 tbsp Stinging Nettle leaves

9. 1 tbsp Irish Sea Moss gel

The instructions are:

1. Get a clean pot, measure 4-6 cups of water or 32-48 ounces of water, and boil it.

2. Add the hard herbs: Pau D'Arco inner bark, peony root, and sarsaparilla root to the boiling water, reduce the heat, and allow it to simmer for at least 25 minutes.

3. Add all the soft herbs: red clover flowers, chaparral leaves, and stems, red raspberry leaves, shepherd's purse, and stinging nettle leaves, and allow it to simmer for an additional 10-15 minutes before turning off the heat.

4. Add the Irish Sea moss gel, and stir it very well before getting a strainer or fine mess or cheesecloth to strain the herbal tea into a cup or jar.

5. The other option is you strain it before adding the Irish Sea moss to the warm herbal tea and stir it very well before consumption.

Administering the Tea

Drink 1 cup 2-3 times per day. But start by taking 1 cup in the morning for the first 3 days of your cleanse, and if your body system tolerates it without any negative effects, you can increase your intake to 2-3 cups per day.

The best time to drink this herbal tea is in the morning on an empty stomach to energize and revitalize your body system and in the evening before going to bed to promote healing during night rest.

Storage and warming of the herbal teas use the same method as the others.

CHAPTER TEN
Herbal Remedy for Lupus
The Cleansing Herbs for Lupus

According to Dr. Sebi, Lupus happens to someone when the central nervous system is compromised because a yeast infection has not been treated properly. Remember that the central nervous system and the immune system are just like one single system as they work simultaneously, and the only way to get rid of Lupus is through intra-cellular cleansing.

The cleansing herbs for Lupus are:

1. Burdock root

2. Cascara Sagrada

3. Chaparral

4. Dandelion

5. Elderberry

6. Mullein

7. Eucalyptus

8. Guaco

9. Rhubarb root

10.   Yellow Dock

11.   Sarsaparilla root

12.   Irish Sea Moss

Because of the need to treat the yeast infection, you will need to add the following herbs (used to treat yeast infection) to your cleansing herbs for Lupus

1. Pau D'Arco

2. Black Walnut

3. Blessed Thistle

4. Bladderwrack

5. Anamu/Guinea Hen weed

How to Cleanse Using the Cleansing Herbs Above to Treat Lupus

To do a detox for the treatment of lupus, you will need to know the following key things:

1. Understanding the cleansing herbal combination for lupus

2. How to prepare and administer the cleansing herbs

3. The storage, warming, and best time to consume the cleansing herbs

Understanding the Cleansing Herbal Combination for Lupus

1. Herbal teas made with burdock root, dandelion flowers, Yellow Dock root, chaparral leaves, and yellow duck root help with the cleansing of the kidney, liver, and blood, which are also important factors to consider when dealing with an autoimmune disease like Lupus.

2. Support digestion and liver health: Herbal teas made with blessed thistle, cascara sagrada bark and rhubarb root has the potency to support digestion and liver health, which is key for lupus treatment.

3. Boost the immune system, repair tissue, and eliminate pathogens: Herbal teas made with Irish Sea moss, anamu, bladderwrack, elderberries, Pau D'Arco bark, chaparral leaves, sarsaparilla root, and black walnut hulls contain properties that are antioxidant, anti-inflammatory, antifungal, and anti-microbial and have the potency to eliminate yeast infection which is the major cause of lupus.

4. Anti-inflammation And Support lungs and respiratory health: Herbal teas made with mullein, eucalyptus, and guaco leaves are very effective remedies for fighting against infection

and respiratory system disorders and reducing inflammation, which is also very important for people suffering from lupus.

How to Prepare and Administer the Cleansing Herbal Teas for Lupus

To cleanse and administer the cleansing herbal teas for Lupus, you will need the following ingredients:

1. tbsp Burdock root (detoxifies the liver, purifies the blood)

2. 1 tbsp Cascara Sagrada bark

3. 1 tbsp Rhubarb root

4. 1 tbsp Yellow Dock root

5. 1 tbsp Sarsaparilla root

6. 1 tbsp Pau D'Arco inner bark

7. 1 tbsp Black Walnut hulls/leaves

8. 1 tbsp Chaparral leaves and stem

9. 1 tbsp Dandelion flowers

10. 1 tbsp Elderberries

11. 1 tbsp Mullein leaves and flowers

12. 1 tbsp Eucalyptus leaves

13. 1 tbsp Guaco leaves

14. 1 tbsp Blessed Thistle leaves, stems, and flowers

15. 1 tbsp Bladderwrack dried fronds or leaves

16. 1 tbsp Anamu (Guinea Hen Weed)

17. 1 tbsp Irish Sea Moss gel

The instructions are:

1. Get a clean pot, measure 6-8 cups of water or 48-64 ounces of water, and boil it.

2. Add all the hard herbs; Burdock root, Cascara Sagrada bark, rhubarb root, yellow dock root,

sarsaparilla root, pau d'arco inner bark, and black walnut hulls or leaves, reduce the heat and allow it to simmer for at least 35 minutes.

3. Add all the soft herbs and the berries: chaparral leaves and stem, dandelion flowers, elderberries, mullein leaves, and flowers, eucalyptus leaves, guaco leaves, blessed thistle, anamu, and bladderwrack and allow it to simmer for another 10-15 minutes before turning off the heat.

4. Get a strainer or fine mesh or cheesecloth and strain the tea into a cup or jar to remove herbal residuals before adding the Irish Sea moss gel.

5. Stir the herbal tea very well for the gel to be completely dissolved before consumption.

Administering the Tea

Drink 1 cup of the herbal cleansing tea twice per day, but you will have to monitor your system to see your tolerance level by drinking one cup per day, for the first 3 days of your cleanse before you can increase it to 2-3 cups per day.

The best time to drink this tea is in the morning before eating anything for optimal detoxification and in the evening before going to bed to support cleansing while the body is enjoying its night's rest.

Just like the other herbal teas, storage and warming are the same thing.

The Revitalizing Herbs for Lupus

The revitalizing herbs for lupus are:

1. Sarsaparilla root

2. Irish Sea Moss

3. Blue Vervain

4. German Chamomile

5. Valerian root

How to Use the Revitalizing Herbs Above to Revitalize the Body System After Cleansing for Lupus?

To revitalize the body system after cleansing for lupus, it is of great importance for you to focus on cleansing the liver, calming the nervous system, boosting the immune system, and managing stress and anxiety. To achieve this, you will need to:

1. Understand the revitalizing herbal combination for lupus

2. How to prepare and administer the herbs

3. The best time to consume the herbs, its storage, and how they can be warmed.

Understanding the Herbal Combination for Revitalizing Lupus

1. Cleanse the liver and blood and reduce inflammation: Herbal teas made with sarsaparilla root help detox the liver and blood and reduce inflammation, which is very important in

revitalizing the body system after cleansing to treat lupus.

2. Digestive health and immune booster: Herbal teas made with Irish Sea moss gel and German Chamomile flowers help revitalize the entire body system by providing 100+ minerals, including calcium, iodine, and potassium, which all have the potency to repair damaged tissue and boost the immune system. German Chamomile flowers also help support digestion and manage stress and anxiety.

3. A calm nervous system supports mental clarity and reduces inflammation and stress: Herbal teas made with blue vervain, German chamomile flowers, and valerian root help to reduce inflammation, promote relaxation, calm the nervous system, reduce stress and anxiety, and support mental clarity. Lastly, valerian root aids

in good sleep, which is all-important for post-cleansing recovery from lupus.

How to Prepare and Administer the Revitalizing Herbs After Cleansing for Lupus

To prepare and administer the revitalizing herbs after cleansing for lupus, you will need the following ingredients:

1. 1 tbsp Sarsaparilla root

2. 1 tbsp Valerian root

3. 1 tbsp Blue Vervain

4. 1 tbsp German Chamomile flowers

5. 1 tbsp Irish Sea Moss gel

The instructions are:

1. Get a clean pot, measure 4-6 cups of water or 32-48 ounces of water, and boil it.

2. Add sarsaparilla and valerian root, reduce the

heat, and allow it to simmer for at least 25 minutes before adding the softer herbs.

3. Add the blue vervain leaves, flowers, and stems, and German chamomile flowers and allow them to simmer for an additional 10-15 minutes before turning off the heat.

4. Get a strainer or cheesecloth to strain the tea into a cup or jar to remove the herbal material.

5. Add the Irish Sea moss gel to the warm tea, and stir it very well until it is completely dissolved.

Administering the Tea

Drink 1 cup of the herbal cleansing tea per day for the first 3 days of the revitalizing period and monitor your system to see your tolerance level before you can increase it to 2-3 cups per day.

The best time to drink this tea is in the morning before eating anything for an energy boost and in the evening before going to bed to promote relaxation and recovery.

Just like the other herbal teas, storage and warming are the same thing.

Don't forget to drink at least a gallon of spring water and get some good sleeping throughout the revitalizing period.

CHAPTER ELEVEN
Herbal Remedy for Strong Bones & Joint
The Cleansing Herbs for Strong Bones & Joint Pain

The cleansing herbs for strong bones and joint pain are:

1. Rhubarb root

2. Prodigiosa

3. Burdock Root

4. Chaparral

5. Dandelion

6. Elderberry

7. Guaco

8. Eucalyptus

9. Mullein

How to Cleanse the Body System Using the Cleansing Herbs Above to Support Strong Bone and Treat Joint Pain?

To do a detox for strong bones and the soothing of joint pain, you will need to know the following key things:

1. Understanding the cleansing herbal combination for supporting strong bones and the treatment of joint pain

2. How to prepare and administer the cleansing herbs

3. The storage, warming, and best time to consume the cleansing herbs

Understanding the Cleansing Herbal Combination for Supporting Strong Bones and Treatment of Joint Pain

1. Anti-inflammation, Antioxidant, and liver support: Herbal teas made with rhubarb root, Prodigiosa leaves, and chaparral are very

137

effective in boosting the liver's health, detoxifying the liver, reducing inflammation related to joints, and regulating blood sugar.

2. Blood purification and boosting of joint health in general: Herbal teas made with burdock root, chaparral, and dandelion help to purify the blood and promote/support joint health. Chaparral aids in the reduction of inflammation, while dandelion helps with the detoxification of the liver and kidneys.

3. Immune booster and respiratory system support: Herbal teas made with elderberries, guaco leaves, and eucalyptus have the potency to boost the immune system, support the respiratory system, and ease inflammation of the joints. Eucalyptus leaves help with the treatment of musculoskeletal pain.

How to Prepare and Administer the Herbal Cleansing Herbs for Strong Bone and Joint Pain

To cleanse and administer the cleansing herbal teas for strong bone and joint pain, you will need the following ingredients:

1. 1 tbsp Rhubarb root

2. 1 tbsp Prodigiosa leaves

3. 1 tbsp Burdock root

4. 1 tbsp Chaparral leaves and stem.

5. 1 tbsp Dandelion flowers, root, and leaves

6. 1 tbsp Elderberries (fresh or dried)

7. 1 tbsp Guaco leaves

8. 1 tbsp Eucalyptus leaves

9. 1 tbsp Mullein leaves and flowers

The instructions are:

1. Get a clean pot, measure 5-6 cups of water or 40-48 ounces of water and boil it.

2. Add cascara Sagrada bark, rhubarb root, burdock root, and chaparral leaves and stems to the boiling water, lower the heat, and allow it to simmer for at least 30 minutes.

3. Add all the softer herbs; Prodigiosa leaves, Dandelion flowers, Guaco leaves, Eucalyptus leaves, and Mullein leaves and flowers, and allow it to simmer for 5 minutes before adding the elderberries.

4. Allow the mixture to simmer for another 10 minutes before turning off the heat.

5. Get a fine mesh or cheesecloth to strain the tea into a cup or jar to separate the plant materials from the herbal tea.

The Administering the Tea

Start by drinking one cup of herbal tea per day for the first three days of your cleanse. Monitor your body's tolerance level before you can increase your intake to 2-3 cups per day.

The best time to drink this herbal tea is in the morning on an empty stomach to boost your energy level and detox the entire body system, and in the evening before going to bed to continue the detoxification while you enjoy a sound night's rest.

Just like all other herbal teas, you can store unused ones in your refrigerator and whenever, you want to consume it, warm it gently using a cooking gas or stove don't microwave your herbal teas.

Don't forget to drink at least a gallon of water per day to support the body in flushing out toxins and lubricating the joints.

Ensure you consume alkaline diets that are calcium-rich to further support bone health while cleansing.

The Revitalizing Herbs for Strong Bone and Joint Pain

The revitalizing herbs for strong bones and joint pain are:

1. Irish Sea moss

2. Horsetail/Shavegrass

3. Dandelion

4. Rhubarb root

5. Bladderwrack

6. Hydrangea

How to Use the Revitalizing Herbs Above to Revitalize the Body System After Cleansing for Strong Bones and Joints?

To revitalize the body system after cleansing for strong bones and joints, you will need to focus on consuming herbal teas that are rich in silica, iodine, calcium, magnesium, potassium, and other nutrients, which are of great importance for strong bones and joints. To achieve this, you will need to know the following:

1. Understand the revitalizing herbal combination for strong bones and joints

2. How to prepare and administer the herbs

3. The best time to consume the herbs, they storage, and how it can be warmed.

Understanding the Herbal Combination for Strong Bones and Joints

1. Support strong bones and joints: Herbal teas that are made with Irish Sea moss gel, dandelion flowers, and rhubarb root are rich in calcium, magnesium, potassium, and other vital minerals that help strengthen bones and support joint health.

2. Formation of collagen and tissue and bone support: Herbal teas made with horsetail, hydrangea, and bladderwrack are very rich in silica, iodine, and other nutrients, which are of

great importance for collagen formation, bone development, joint function, reduced calcifications, and strengthening of bones and connective tissue.

How to Prepare and Administer the Revitalizing Herbs after Cleansing for Strong Bones and Joints?

To prepare and administer the revitalizing herbs after cleansing for strong bones and joints, you will need the following ingredients:

1. 1 tbsp Rhubarb root

2. 1 tbsp Hydrangea root and rhizome

3. 1 tbsp Horsetail (Shavegrass) aerial parts

4. 1 tbsp Dandelion flowers

5. 1 tbsp Bladderwrack leaves, stems, and air bladders

6. 2 tbsp Irish Sea Moss gel

The instructions are:

1. Get a clean pot, measure 5-6 cups of water, or 40-48 ounces of water and boil it.

2. Add rhubarb root and hydrangea root/rhizome to the boiling water, reduce the heat, and allow it to simmer for at least 30 minutes.

3. Add the bladderwrack leaves/stems/air bladders, and horsetail aerial parts, and allow the mixture to simmer for an additional 10 minutes.

4. Add the dandelion flowers to the simmering mixture and allow it to simmer for an additional 5-10 minutes.

5. Get a fine mesh, strainer, or cheesecloth to strain the tea into a cup or jar to remove the herbal residual.

6. Add the Irish sea moss gel to the warm herbal tea and stir it very well until the gel is completely dissolved.

Administering the Tea

Start by drinking one cup of herbal tea per day for the first three days of your revitalizing process and make sure you monitor your system tolerance level before you can increase your intake to 2-3 cups per day.

The best time to drink this herbal tea is in the morning on an empty stomach or between meals to boost your energy level and detox the entire body system, and in the evening before going to bed to continue with the nourishing and revitalizing of the bone and joint health while you rest.

Just like all other herbal teas, you can store unused ones in your refrigerator, and whenever you want to consume it, warm it gently using a cooking gas or stove. Don't microwave your herbal teas. And don't store herbal teas for more than 3 days.

CHAPTER TWELVE
Herbal Remedy for Thyroid Disorder
The Cleansing Herbs for Under or Overactive Thyroid (Hypo and Hyper)

The cleansing herbs for under or overactive thyroid (hypo and hyper) are:

1. Cascara Sagrada

2. Rhubarb root

3. Prodigiosa

4. Burdock root

5. Chaparral

6. Dandelion

7. Elderberry

8. Guaco

9. Eucalyptus

10.   Mullein

How to Cleanse the Body System Using the Cleansing Herbs Above for Thyroid Disorders?

To do a detox for thyroid disorders, you will need to know the following key things:

1. Understanding the cleansing herbal combination for thyroid disorders.

2. How to prepare and administer the cleansing herbs

3. The storage, warming, and best time to consume the cleansing herbs

Understanding the Cleansing Herbal Combination for Thyroid Disorders

1. Support digestion and general cleansing of the body: Herbal teas made with cascara Sagrada bark, chaparral, and guaco leaves stimulate digestion and bowel movement, aiding in detoxification, which is essential for thyroid health, and guaco still contains anti-

inflammation properties that help with reducing inflammation.

2. Sugar regulation and hormonal balance: Teas made with dandelion and prodigiosa leaves help to regulate blood sugar and support both kidney and liver functions, which are essential for maintaining balanced hormone levels.

3. Detox and support thyroid functionalities: Herbal teas made with burdock root, chaparral leaves, and stem are rich in detoxifying properties that help to cleanse the liver, and blood, and regulate hormonal production, which supports thyroid functionalities.

4. Anti-inflammation And immune system support: Herbal teas made with elderberries and guaco is very effective in boosting the immune system, cleansing the entire biological body, and reducing inflammation, which is crucial for

thyroid health.

5. Support respiratory and thyroid health and combat infection: Herbal teas made with mullein, guaco, and eucalyptus leaves are very rich in anti-inflammatory and antimicrobial properties that help combat infections, and support and detoxify the thyroid and respiratory system.

How to Prepare and Administer Cleansing Herbs for Thyroid Disorders?

To prepare and administer the cleansing herbs for thyroid disorders, you will need the following ingredients:

1. 1 tbsp Cascara Sagrada bark

2. 1 tbsp Rhubarb root

3. 1 tbsp Burdock root

4. 1 tbsp Prodigiosa leaves

5. 1 tbsp Chaparral leaves and stem

6. 1 tbsp Dandelion flowers

7. 1 tbsp fresh or dried Elderberries

8. 1 tbsp Guaco leaves

9. 1 tbsp Eucalyptus leaves

10.   1 tbsp Mullein leaves and flowers

The instructions are:

1. Get a clean pot, measure 5-6 cups of water, or 40-48 ounces of water, and boil it.

2. Add all the hard herbs: cascara Sagrada bark, rhubarb root, and burdock root to the boiling water lower the heat, and allow it to simmer for at least 25 minutes.

3. Add the Elderberries and allow it to simmer for 5 minutes before adding all the softer herbs.

4. Add prodigiosa leaves, chaparral leaves/stem, dandelion flowers, guaco leaves, eucalyptus leaves, and Mullein leaves/flowers, and allow it to simmer for an additional 10-15 minutes before turning off the heat.

5. Get a strainer or fine mesh/cheesecloth to strain the tea into a cup or jar to remove the plant material from the herbal tea.

Administering the Tea:

Start by drinking one cup of herbal tea per day for the first three days of your cleansing period and ensure you monitor your system tolerance level before you can increase your intake to 2-3 cups per day.

The best time to drink this herbal tea is in the morning on an empty stomach or between meals to boost your energy level and detox the entire body system, in the evening before going to bed to continue with the cleaning while you have a sweet night's rest.

Just like all other herbal teas, you can store unused ones in your refrigerator, and whenever you want to consume it, warm it gently using a cooking gas or stove. Don't microwave your herbal teas. And don't store herbal teas for more than 3 days.

The Revitalizing Herbs for Under or Overactive Thyroid (Hypo and Hyper)

The revitalizing herbs for under or overactive thyroid (hypo and hyper) are:

1. Irish sea moss

2. Kalawalla

3. Bladderwrack

4. Bugleweed

5. Blue Vervain

6. Valerian root

7. German Chamomile

How to Use the Revitalizing Herbs Above to Revitalize the Body System After Cleansing for Thyroid Disorders?

To revitalize the body system after cleansing for thyroid disorder, you will need to focus on consuming herbal teas that have the potency to cleanse the entire body system, regulate your sugar and hormone levels, support the thyroid system, boost the immune system, and enhance respiratory functionality. To achieve this, you will need to know the following:

1. Understand the revitalizing herbal combination for thyroid disorders

2. How to prepare and administer the herbs

3. The best time to consume the herbs, its storage, and how they can be warmed.

Understanding the Revitalizing Herbal Combination for Thyroid Disorders

1. Stress management and calming of the nervous system: Herbal teas made with Valerian root and

German chamomile have rich properties that help calm the nervous system, reduce stress and anxiety, and support sound sleep. Lastly, valerian root also helps the body to recover quickly from thyroid disorders.

2. Essential nutrients needed by the body and immune booster: Herbal teas made with Irish Sea moss, Bladderwrack, and kalawalla are very effective in supporting the immune system and provide the body with over 100+ nutrients, including iodine and other essential nutrients that help with the treatment of thyroid disorders and replenish the body system.

3. Hormone regulator: Herbal teas made with Bugleweed and Bladderwrack help to produce thyroid hormone and also regulate its production.

How to Prepare and Administer the Revitalizing Herbal Teas after Cleansing for Thyroid Disorders?

To prepare and administer the revitalizing herbal teas after cleansing for thyroid disorders, you will need the following ingredients:

1. 1 tbsp Irish Sea Moss gel

2. 1 tbsp Kalawalla rhizome

3. 1 tbsp Bladderwrack

4. 1 tbsp Bugleweed aerial parts

5. 1 tbsp Blue Vervain

6. 1 tbsp Valerian root

7. 1 tbsp German Chamomile flowers

The instructions are:

1. Get a clean pot, measure 5-6 cups of water, or 40-48 ounces of water, and boil it.

2. Add the hard herbs: Kalawalla rhizome, Bladderwrack, and Valerian root to the boiling water, reduce the heat, and let it simmer for at least 20 minutes.

3. Add Bugleweed and Blue Vervain to the pot with the mixture and allow it to simmer for an additional 10 minutes before adding the softer herbs.

4. Add German Chamomile flowers and Irish Sea Moss gel to the mixture, stir, and allow it to simmer for an additional 5 minutes before turning off the heat.

5. Get a strainer or fine mesh or cheesecloth to strain the tea into a cup or jar to remove herbal residual.

Administering the Tea

Start by consuming 1 cup per day for the first 3 days

before adding your consumption to 2 cups per day. Ensure you monitor your tolerance level before increasing the dose.

The best time to drink this herbal tea is in the morning before meal for the first three days, before drinking it in the morning and evening before going to bed for replenishing relaxation.

The storage and reheating of the herbal tea process is the same as other herbal teas.

CHAPTER THIRTEEN
Herbal Remedy for Skin Disease
Cleansing Herbs for Skin Diseases

The cleansing herbs for skin diseases are:

1. Guaco

2. Dandelion

3. Burdock root

4. Sarsaparilla

5. Mullein

6. Chaparral

7. Cascara Sagrada

8. Elderberry

9. Irish sea moss

How to Cleanse the Body System Using the Cleansing Herbs Above for Skin Diseases?

To do a detox for skin diseases, you will need to know

the following key things:

1. Understanding the cleansing herbal combination for skin diseases.

2. How to prepare and administer the cleansing herbs

3. The storage, warming, and best time to consume the cleansing herbs

Understanding the Cleansing Herbal Combination for Skin Disease.

1. Anti-inflammation and general cleansing: Herbal teas made with guaco, dandelion, and mullein are known for their powerful properties that help to reduce inflammation and cleanse the entire body system, which helps to resolve underlying skin issues.

2. Cleansing of the blood and neutralizing free radicals: Herbal teas made with Chaparral leaves and stem Sarsaparilla root and burdock root are

known for the effective properties that they contain, which help to purify the blood, neutralize free radicals that contribute to skin irritation and imbalance, and reduce skin damage such as acne, eczema, etc.

3. Immune booster and minerals replenishment: Herbal teas made with Irish Sea moss and elderberries contain over 100+ minerals that the body needs to stay healthy, and they boost the immune system, helping the body to naturally clear skin irritants and repair damaged skin.

How to Prepare and Administer the Cleansing Herbal Teas for Skin Diseases?

To prepare and administer the cleansing herbal teas for skin diseases, you will need the following ingredients:

1. 1 tbsp Guaco leaves

2. 1 tbsp Dandelion flowers

3. 1 tbsp Burdock root

4. 1 tbsp Sarsaparilla root

5. 1 tbsp Mullein leaves and flowers

6. 1 tbsp Chaparral leaves and stem

7. 1/2 tbsp Cascara Sagrada bark

8. 1 tbsp Elderberries

9. 1 tbsp Irish Sea Moss gel

The instructions are:

1. Get a clean pot and measure 5-6 cups of water or 40-48 ounces of water and boil it.

2. Add all the hard herbs: Burdock root, Sarsaparilla root, Chaparral leaves and stem, and Cascara Sagrada bark. Reduce the heat and allow it to simmer for at least 20 minutes.

3. Add Guaco leaves and Mullein leaves to the mixture and allow it to simmer for an additional 10 minutes.

4. Add the dandelion flowers and elderberries and allow it to simmer for an additional 5-10 minutes before removing the pot from heat.

5. Add Irish sea moss gel to the warm herbal mixture, and stir very well to dissolve into the tea mixture.

6. Get a strainer or fine mesh or cheesecloth to strain the tea into a cup or jar to remove the herbal materials.

Administering the Tea

Drink 1 cup of the herbal tea per day for the first 3 days of your cleanse and monitor your tolerance level before you can increase it to 2-3 cups per day if your system tolerates it.

The best time to drink this tea is in the morning on an empty stomach or between meals to maximize absorption and detox effects for the first 3 days and before going to bed when you have increased your intake.

Storage and heating, it's the same thing with other herbal teas.

Ensure you get enough rest to manage your stress, as skin conditions often worsen with much stress.

The Revitalizing Herbs After Cleansing for Skin Diseases

The revitalizing herbs after cleansing for skin diseases are:

1. Sarsaparilla root

2. Irish Sea Moss

3. Blue Vervain

4. German Chamomile

5. Valerian root

6. Red clover

How to Use the Revitalizing Herbs Above to Revitalize the Body System After Cleansing for Skin Diseases?

To revitalize the body system after cleansing for skin disease, you will need to focus on getting more rest, calming the nervous and respiratory systems, regulating your sugar and hormone levels, supporting the thyroid system, and boosting the immune system. To achieve this, you will need to know the following:

1. Understand the revitalizing herbal combination for skin diseases

2. How to prepare and administer the herbs

3. The best time to consume the herbs, its storage, and how they can be warmed.

Understand the Revitalizing Herbal Combination for Skin Diseases

Every herb in revitalizing the body for skin disease has a particular function that makes it to be included as part of the herbs for skin diseases.

1. For the need to detox or purify the blood, and skin, and boosts skin health, sarsaparilla root, and red clover were included as part of the revitalizing herbs.

2. The need to boost the immune system and replenish all the lost nutrients due to skin diseases and cleanse the system, to aid healthy skin, Irish Sea Moss gel is included.

3. To calm the nervous system, manage stress, reduce inflammation, and repair damaged skin, blue Vervain and German Chamomile flowers are the best herbs for skin conditions.

4. Regulation of hormones: Red Clover flowers are an effective herb for the detoxification of blood that aids in supporting skin health and regulating hormones.

How to Prepare and Administer the Revitalizing Herbs for Revitalizing of the Body System After Cleansing for Skin Diseases?

To prepare and administer the revitalizing herbs after cleansing for skin diseases, you will need the following ingredients:

1. 1 tbsp of Sarsaparilla root,

2. 1 tbsp of Blue Vervain leaves and flowers

3. 1 tbsp of German Chamomile flower

4. 1 tbsp of Valerian root

5. 1 tbsp of Red Clover flowers

6. 1 tbsp of Irish Sea Moss gel

The instructions are:

1. Get a clean pot and measure 5-6 cups of water or 40-48 ounces of water and boil it.

2. Add Sarsaparilla root and Valerian root, reduce

the heat, and allow it to simmer for at least 25 minutes.

3. Add Red Clover flowers, Blue Vervain leaves and flowers, and German Chamomile flower, and allow it to simmer for an additional 10 minutes.

4. Get a strainer or fine mesh or cheesecloth to strain the tea into a cup or jar to remove the herbal residual.

5. As the herbal tea is still hot, add the Irish Sea moss gel and stir it properly until it completely dissolves.

The administration:

Drink 1 cup of the herbal tea in the morning on an empty stomach and 1 cup in about an hour in the evening before going to bed to nourish and revitalize the body after the cleansing process.

Please note that the same method applies for storage and reheating of the unused herbal teas.

Herbs Used as Poultice, Skin Wash Paste, or Decoctions

The herbs used for poultice, skin wash, paste, or decoction for skin diseases are:

1. Burdock root paste: This tropical skin treatment is used all over the globe for the treatment of skin diseases like Acne, abscesses, carbuncle, eczema, and psoriasis. To create a burdock root paste, grind the dried burdock root and mix it with olive oil. Apply it directly to the affected areas for 20-30 minutes before rinsing it off with warm water.

2. Red Clover infusion is a topical skin treatment that can be applied to the skin for the treatment of skin diseases such as cancer, eczema, and psoriasis, etc.

To prepare the red clover infusion, get a cup of dried Red Clover flowers and a cup of olive oil. Place the dried Red Clover flowers in a glass jar, pour the oil into it, cover the herbs completely, seal the jar, and leave it in a warm, sunny spot for at least 4 weeks, shaking it daily. After this duration, get fine clothes or a strainer to strain the oil. Apply the oil directly to the affected areas for an excellent result.

3. Dandelion leaves or root paste: either of the pastes is very rich in vitamins, minerals, and antioxidants that help to combat and reduce inflammation and heal skin conditions such as Eczema and psoriasis, etc. To prepare dandelion leaves or root paste, get a handful of fresh dandelion leaves or roots or the dried leaves or root powder of dandelion, grind or crush the fresh or dried dandelion leaves or roots, and mix it with a little water to create a paste. Apply the paste directly to all the affected skin areas and

leave it for 20–30 minutes before rinsing it off with warm water.

4. Juniper berry can also be applied topically to treat skin ailments and conditions. It is used to treat conditions like acne, athlete's foot, fungi infections, warts, skin growths, cystitis, psoriasis, and eczema. To prepare Juniper berries, get a handful or ¼ cup of dried Juniper berries and a cup of olive oil, grind the dried Juniper berries, and pour them into a clean glass jar. Pour the 1 cup of olive oil to cover all the ground juniper berries, seal the jar, and leave it in a warm spot for at least 4 weeks, shaking it every day for the 4 weeks. Get a strainer and strain the oil. Apply the oil directly to all the affected skin 1–2 times daily.

5. Irish Sea moss gel aids in curing various skin diseases such as Eczema, psoriasis, sunburn,

varicose veins, rashes, and dermatitis, and can also help to soothe and hydrate the skin and reduce skin inflammation. To prepare the Irish sea moss gel, get fresh or dried, raw Irish Sea Moss and spring water. Rinse the sea moss to remove any sand or debris and soak it in the spring water for at least 12 hours until it completely softens and expands. Once it is softened and expanded, blend it with enough spring water to cover the sea moss until it forms a smooth, gel-like consistency. Apply it directly to all the affected areas and leave it for 20–30 minutes before rinsing off with warm water.

6. Guaco ointment with the leaves can be used externally for the treatment of pruritus, wounds, neuralgia, eczema, and rheumatic pain. To prepare Guaco decoction, get fresh guaco leaves, grind or crush them, and mix them with a small amount of olive oil to form a smooth paste. Heat

the paste gently on low heat for at least 5 minutes to infuse the oil with its medicinal properties. Apply the ointment 1-2 times to the affected areas as soon as it gets cool.

7. Pau D'Arco poultice using the bark can be used to treat fungal infection, hemorrhoids, wounds, eczema, and skin inflammation. To prepare Pau D'Arco poultice, grind or crush Pau D'Arco bark, and mix it in warm water to form a thick paste. Apply the paste directly to all the affected areas of the skin, bandage it and leave it on for at least 20 minutes before rinsing it off with lukewarm water.

8. Eucalyptus steam treatment aids in reducing skin inflammation, repels insects and treats dry skin and wounds from acne, eczema, and psoriasis. To do this, get a handful of fresh or dried eucalyptus leaves, boil 2-3 liters of water, and

add the handful of eucalyptus leaves. Turn off the heat and allow the leaves to steep for about 10 minutes. Get a stool, lean over the pot, cover your head with a duvet or blanket to trap the steam, and allow the steam to penetrate your skin for at least 8 minutes before rinsing your face or affected skin area with cool water and pat dry. Do this routine, 2–3 times per week, to treat skin diseases and promote clear skin.

9. Pavana is used to treat boils and other skin lesions. It is also typically used to treat skin conditions such as itching, scabies, eczema, and rashes. To create pavana paste, grind, or crush pavana into a powder mix it with olive oil and stir it well for 1-2 minutes to create a thick, spreadable paste. You can apply it directly to all the affected areas of the skin. You do not need to let the mixture to sit for a long time before use. You can leave the paste on the skin for 20–

30 minutes before rinsing it off with warm water.

10.   Sage relieves and improves annoying skin conditions such as acne, athlete's foot, and changed skin and relieves symptoms of eczema and psoriasis. To use Sage, kindly infuse the Sage leaves into olive oil for at least 6 hours and apply it to affected areas for an excellent result. Use the infusion to gently wash the affected skin, or get a clean cloth, soak it in the infusion, and apply it as a compress to all the affected skin areas. Leave the compress on for 10–15 minutes, before rinsing the affected areas of the skin with cool water. Do this routine every night before sleeping or morning when you wake up and the night before going to bed.

11.   Draco known as dragon's blood is commonly used to treat vaginal infections, hemorrhoids, and skin conditions such as

eczema, as well as for insect bites and stings. It is also widely used to aid in the acceleration of healing wounds. To prepare Draco's infusion, get 1 tablespoon of Draco's resin boil 2 cups of hot water, and pour the Draco's resin before removing it from heat immediately. Allow it to steep for at least 10 minutes before straining it. Use the infusion 1-2 times daily to wash the affected skin or soak a clean cloth. Apply it as a compress on all the affected areas and leave it for at least 10 minutes.

CHAPTER FOURTEEN
Herbal Remedy for Heart Disorders
The Cleansing Herbs for Healing Heart Disorders.

The cleansing herbs for healing heart disorders such as heart failure, palpitation, and enhancing the heart's general functionalities are:

1. Cascara Sagrada

2. Rhubarb root

3. Prodigiosa

4. Burdock root

5. Chaparral

6. Dandelion

7. Elderberry

8. Guaco

9. Eucalyptus

10.   Mullein

How to Cleanse the Body System Using the Cleansing Herbs Above for Heart Disorders?

To do a detox for heart disorders, you will need to know the following key things:

1. Understanding the cleansing herbal combination for heart disorders

2. How to prepare and administer the cleansing herbs

3. The storage, warming, and best time to consume the cleansing herbs

Understanding the cleansing herbal combination for heart disorders

1. Support liver and digestive health and toxin elimination: Herbal teas made with cascara sagrada bark and rhubarb root have properties that have the potency to help eliminate toxins, stimulate gentle bowel cleansing, and support

178

the liver and digestive health. Aside from other functions, prodigiosa and burdock root also help to enhance liver function.

2. Cleanse blood and regulate blood sugar level: Herbal tea made with prodigiosa, and burdock root helps to detoxify the blood and regulate blood sugar. Additionally, burdock root helps enhance both liver and kidney health and promotes circulation.

3. Antioxidant, anti-inflammation, and respiratory system support: Herbal teas made with chaparral, elderberry, and eucalyptus leaves are very effective in treating free radicals, supporting respiratory health, reducing inflammation, and supporting circulation, which is very crucial to the heart's health.

4. Immune support and cholesterol regulation: Herbal teas made with dandelion and

elderberries are very potent in boosting the immune system, boosting the immune system, and enhancing heart health.

How to Prepare and Administer the Cleansing Herbal Teas for Heart Disorders?

To prepare and administer the herbal cleansing tea for heart disease, you will need the following ingredients:

1. 1 tbsp of Cascara Sagrada bark

2. 1 tbsp of Rhubarb root

3. Prodigiosa leaves

4. 1 tbsp of Burdock root

5. 1 tbsp of Chaparral leaves/stem

6. Dandelion flowers

7. Elderberry

8. 1 tbsp of Guaco leaves

9. Eucalyptus leaves

10. Mullein leaves and flowers

The preparations are:

1. Get a clean pot, measure 5-6 cups of water or 40-48 ounces of water and boil it.

2. Add cascara Sagrada bark, rhubarb root, and burdock root to the boiling water. Reduce the heat and allow it to simmer for at least 25 minutes.

3. Add Dandelion flowers, Prodigiosa leaves, Mullein leaves/flowers, Elderberry, and Eucalyptus leaves, and let the mixture simmer for 10-15 minutes before straining it.

4. Get a strainer, fine mesh, or cheesecloth to strain the tea into a cup or jar to remove the herbal residual.

Administering the Tea

Drink 2-3 cups of the herbal tea per day. For the first 3 days of your cleanse, drink 1-2 cups and monitor your tolerance level before you can increase to 2-3 cups per day if your system tolerates it.

The best time to drink this tea is in the morning on an empty stomach or between meals to maximize absorption and detox effects for the first 3 days and before going to bed when you have increased your intake.

Storage and heating, it's the same thing with other herbal teas.

The Revitalizing Herbs for Healing Heart Disorders After Cleansing for Heart Disorders

The revitalizing herbs for healing heart disorders, such as heart failure, palpitation, and heart attack, and enhancing the heart's general functionalities, are:

1. Lily of the Valley

2. Irish Sea moss

3. Hawthorn Berry

4. Sarsaparilla root

5. Olive leaf extract

6. Condurango

7. Flor de Manita

8. Bugleweed

9. Fennel

10.   Organic Kelp

11.   Elderberry

12.   Flor de Tila

13.   Shepherds purse

How to Use the Revitalizing Herbs Above to Revitalize the Body System After Cleansing for Heart Disorders?

To revitalize the body system after cleansing for heart disorders, you need to focus on getting more rest, calming the nervous system, supporting circulation, regulating sugar levels, boosting cardiovascular health, reducing inflammation, boosting the immune system, etc. To achieve this, you will need to know the following:

1. Understand the revitalizing herbal combination for heart disorders

2. How to prepare and administer the herbs

3. The best time to consume the herbs, its storage, and how they can be warmed.

Understand the Revitalizing Herbal Combination for Heart Disorders

1. Support cardiovascular health: Herbal teas made with whole kelp plants, olive leaf extract, and lily

of the valley are generally known for their functions in supporting cardiovascular health and heart rhythm, and kelp and olive leaf extract also have some minerals and antioxidant properties that help with supporting metabolism.

2. Immune booster, tissue repairs, and replenishing of lost nutrients: Herbal teas made with Irish Sea moss, condurango, and elderberry contain lots of minerals and antioxidants that help to boost the immune system and blood circulation and also aid in the repair of damaged tissue and replenish lost nutrients that the body might have lost due to the cleansing or the effect of the disease.

3. Purifies blood, lowers blood pressure, and enhances circulation: Herbal teas made with Hawthorn berry, sarsaparilla root, condurango,

Shepherd's Purse, and Flor de Tila flower help to purify the blood, lower blood pressure, enhance circulation, calm the nervous system, reduces tension, and continue with the cleansing to cleans what is left after cleansing, etc.

4. Anti-inflammation, calming the nervous system, and supports digestion: Herbal teas made with Fennel seed, floor de tila, and bugleweed are very effective in reducing inflammation, calming the nervous system, supporting digestion, and circulation, reducing tension, and regulating the heart rate which directly or indirectly benefits heart health.

How to Prepare and Administer the Revitalizing Herbal Teas for Heart Disorders?

To prepare and administer the herbal revitalizing tea for heart disease after you cleansing for heart disorders, you will need the following ingredients:

1. ½ tbsp of Lily of the Valley flowers

2. 1 tbsp of Irish Sea Moss gel

3. 1 tbsp of Hawthorn Berry

4. 1 tbsp of Sarsaparilla root

5. ½ tbsp of Olive leaf extract

6. 1 tbsp of Condurango bark

7. 2 tbsp of Flor de Manita flowers

8. 1 tbsp of Bugleweed aerial parts

9. 2 tbsp of Fennel seed

10.   2 tbsp of Whole Kelp plant

11.   2 tbsp of Elderberry

12.   2 tbsp of Flor de Tila flower

13.   2 tbsp of Shepherd's Purse aerial parts

The instructions are:

1. Get a clean pot, measure 5-6 cups of water, or 40-48 ounces of water, and boil it.

2. Once the water is boiling, add Sarsaparilla root and Condurango bark, reduce the heat, and allow it to simmer for at least 20 minutes.

3. Add fennel seed, whole kelp, Hawthorn Berry, Shepherd's Purse, Bugleweed, and elderberry, and allow it to simmer for another 5-10 minutes.

4. Add Flor de Manita, Flor de Tila, and Lily of the Valley and allow it to simmer for another 10 minutes.

5. Get a strainer, fine mesh, or cheesecloth and strain the tea into a cup or jar to remove the herbal extract.

6. While the tea is still warm, add Irish Sea moss gel and Olive leaf extract, and stir it properly until it is completely dissolved.

Administration

Drink 2 cups per day: 1 in the morning and the other 1 cup in the evening. Always ensure you monitor your tolerance level before you can increase the intake to 2-3 cups per day.

The best time to drink this tea is in the morning on an empty stomach or between meals to help with the balancing of minerals, antioxidants, and specific heart-supportive compounds that help to restore energy and resilience to the cardiovascular system, and before going to bed to have a sound rest at night while the body replenishes all its lost nutrients.

Storage and heating, it's the same thing with other herbal teas.

CHAPTER FIFTEEN
Herbal Remedy for Cancer
The Cleansing Herbs to Treat All Types of Cancer

The cleansing herbs to treat all types of cancer are:

1. Cascara Sagrada

2. Rhubarb root

3. Prodigiosa

4. Burdock root

5. Chaparral

6. Dandelion

7. Elderberry

8. Guaco

9. Eucalyptus

10.   Mullein

How to Cleanse the Body System Using the Cleansing Herbs Above for Cancer?

To do a detox for cancer, you will need to know the following key things:

1. Understanding the cleansing herbal combination for cancer

2. How to prepare and administer the cleansing herbs

3. The storage, warming, and best time to consume the cleansing herbs

Understanding the Cleansing Herbal Combination for Cancer

1. Stimulate digestion and act as a laxative: herbal teas made with Cascara Sagrada bark and Rhubarb root are rich in laxative properties that aid in relaxation, stimulate digestion, and promote cleansing and elimination of toxins, which are key for eliminating cancer.

2. Anti-inflammation, antimicrobial, and antioxidants: Herbal teas made with eucalyptus leaves, elderberry, Guaco leaves, chaparral, and mullein are rich in anti-inflammation, antimicrobial, and antioxidant properties that have the potency to reduce inflammation, neutralize free radicals, and promote gentle detoxification, which is key to eradicating cancer.

3. Reduce oxidative stress, purify the blood, kidney, and liver: Herbal teas made with rhubarb root, Prodigiosa, burdock root, and dandelion have the potency to reduce oxidative stress, purify the blood, kidney, liver, and balance blood sugar levels.

4. Enhance the respiratory system: Herbal teas made with guaco, mullein, and eucalyptus help to boost and enhance the functionalities of the respiratory system, which is key to the

elimination of cancer.

How to Prepare and Administer the Cleansing Herbal Teas for Cancer?

To prepare and administer the herbal cleansing tea for cancer, you will need the following ingredients:

1. 1 tbsp of Cascara Sagrada

2. 1 tbsp of Rhubarb root

3. 1 tbsp of Prodigiosa leaves

4. 1 tbsp of Burdock root

5. 1 tbsp of Chaparral leaves and stem

6. 1 tbsp of dandelion flowers

7. 1 tbsp of Elderberries

8. 1 tbsp of guaco leaves

9. 1 tbsp of eucalyptus leaves

10.   1 tbsp of mullein leaves/flowers

The instructions are:

1. Get a clean pot, measure 5-6 cups of water, or 40-48 ounces of water, and boil it.

2. Once the water is boiling, add Burdock root, Rhubarb root, and Cascara Sagrada, reduce the heat, and allow it to simmer for at least 20 minutes.

3. Add chaparral and elderberries, and allow it to simmer for an additional 10 minutes before adding the other softer herbs.

4. Add prodigiosa, guaco, dandelion flowers, mullein, and Eucalyptus to the mixture and allow it to simmer for an additional 10 minutes.

5. Get a fine mesh, or cheesecloth and strain the tea into a cup or jar to remove the herbal residual.

Administration

Drink 2 cups daily. That is, one cup in the morning

and 1 cup in the evening to assess your tolerance level to decide if you can increase your intake to 2-3 cups per day.

The best time to take this herbal tea is in the morning and evening.

The storage and reheating of the herbal tea is the same as other herbal teas.

The Revitalizing Herbs to Revitalize the Body System After Cleansing for Cancer

The revitalizing herbs to treat all types of cancer are:

1. Contribo

2. Cordoncillo Negro

3. Kalawalla

4. Pavana

5. Sarsaparilla

6. Irish Sea moss

How to Use the Revitalizing Herbs Above to Revitalize the Body System After Cleansing to Eliminate the Root Cause of Cancer?

To revitalize the body system after cleansing the body system to eliminate the root cause of cancer, there is a need to focus on reducing inflammation, immune modulation, cellular rejuvenation, neutralizing free radicals, energizing the body, tissue repair, etc.

To achieve this, you will need to know the following:

1. Understand the revitalizing herbal combination to eliminate the root cause of cancer

2. How to prepare and administer the herbs

3. The best time to consume the herbs, its storage, and how they can be warmed.

Understand the Revitalizing Herbal Combination to Eliminate the Root-cause of Cancer

1. Replenish essential nutrients and energy booster:

Herbal teas made with contribo root and Irish Sea moss are very effective in providing the body with the essential nutrients needed for tissue repair, hydration, and energy, enhancing speedy recovery and overall vitality.

2. Anti-inflammation, Antioxidant, and immune booster: Herbal teas made with Cordoncillo Negro leaves, Kalawalla rhizome, Sarsaparilla root, and pavana are very effective in reducing inflammation, immune modulation, cellular rejuvenation, neutralizing free radicals, etc., which are all important in revitalizing the body system to eliminate cancer.

How to Prepare and Administer the Revitalizing Herbs After Cleansing to Eliminate the Root Cause of Cancer

To prepare and administer the revitalizing herbs after cleansing to eliminate the root cause of cancer, you will need the following ingredients:

1. 1 tbsp of Contribo root/stems

2. 1 tbsp of Cordoncillo Negro leaves

3. 1 tbsp of Kalawalla rhizome

4. 1 tbsp of Pavana root/leaves

5. 1 tbsp of Sarsaparilla root

6. 1-2 tbsp of Irish sea moss gel.

The instructions are:

1. Get a clean pot, measure 6-8 cups of water or 48-64 ounces of water, and boil it

2. Once the water is boiling, add Contribo root/stems, Kalawalla rhizome, and sarsaparilla root, reduce the heat and allow it to simmer for at least 25 minutes.

3. Add Cordoncillo Negro and pavana leaves and allow it to simmer for another 10 minutes before turning off the heat.

4. Get a strainer, fine mesh, or cheesecloth and strain the tea into a cup or jar to remove the herbal extract.

5. While the tea is still warm, add the Irish Sea moss gel and stir it properly until it is completely dissolved.

Administration

Start by drinking 1 cup per day for the first three days of your revitalization before you can increase it to 2 cups daily: 1 cup in the morning and the other 1 cup in the evening to help support long-term revitalization and mineral replenishment.

Storage and reheating are the same as other herbal teas.

CHAPTER SIXTEEN
Herbal Remedy for Anemia
The cleansing Herbs for the Treatment of Anemia

The cleansing herbs for the treatment of anemia are:

1. Cascara Sagrada

2. Rhubarb Root

3. Prodigiosa

4. Burdock Root

5. Chaparral

6. Dandelion

7. Elderberry

8. Guaco

9. Eucalyptus

10. Mullein

How to Cleanse the Body System Using the Cleansing Herbs Above for Anemia?

To do a detox for anemia, you will need to know the following key things:

1. Understanding the cleansing herbal combination for anemia

2. How to prepare and administer the cleansing herbs

3. The storage, warming, and best time to consume the cleansing herbs

Understanding the Cleansing Herbal Combination for Anemia

1. Support digestion, liver functions, and the elimination of toxins: Herbal teas made with Cascara Sagrada bark, Rhubarb root, burdock root, and Prodigiosa leaves are very effective in supporting the digestive system, liver functions, and the elimination of toxins. Prodigiosa also helps the body to absorb nutrients, while

burdock roots purify the blood.

2. Anti-inflammation, and support kidney and liver: Herbal teas made with Chaparral leaves/stem, guaco, and dandelion help reduce inflammation, neutralize free radicals, and support kidney and liver function.

3. Support blood, immune, and respiratory systems and cleansing of the respiratory system: Herbal teas made with mullein, eucalyptus, and elderberry help support respiratory health, boost the immune system, and calm inflammation with their inflammatory and antioxidant properties.

How to Prepare and Administer Cleansing Herbal Teas to Eliminate the Root Cause of Anemia?

To prepare and administer herbal cleansing tea to eliminate the root cause of anemia, you will need the following ingredients:

1. 1 tbsp of Cascara Sagrada bark

2. 1 tbsp of Rhubarb Root

3. 1 tbsp of Prodigiosa leaves

4. 1 tbsp of Burdock Root

5. 1 tbsp of Chaparral leaves and stem

6. 1 tbsp of Dandelion flowers

7. 1 tbsp of fresh/dried elderberry

8. 1 tbsp of Guaco leaves

9. 1 tbsp of Eucalyptus leaves

10.   1 tbsp of Mullein leaves and flowers

The Instructions are:

1. Get a clean pot, measure 6-8 cups of water or 48-64 ounces of water, and boil it

2. Once the water is boiling, add Cascara Sagrada bark, Burdock Root, and Rhubarb Root, reduce

the heat, and allow it to simmer for at least 20 minutes.

3. Add elderberry, and Chaparral leaves and stem and allow it to simmer for an additional 5-10 minutes before adding the other softer herbs.

4. Add prodigiosa leaves, dandelion flowers, guaco leaves, eucalyptus leaves, and mullein leaves and flowers, and allow it to simmer for an additional 10-15 minutes before turning off the heat.

5. Get a fine mesh, or cheesecloth and strain the tea into a cup or jar to remove the herbal extract.

Administration of the tea

Start by drinking 1 cup per day. Monitor your tolerance level for the first 3 days before you decide to increase your intake to 2 cups per day.

The best time to take this herbal tea is in the morning before breakfast and at night before going to bed.

Storage of the herbal teas leftover and reheating are the same as the other herbal teas.

The Revitalizing Herbs After Cleansing for the Treatment of Anemia

The revitalizing herbs after cleansing for the treatment of anemia are:

1. Sarsaparilla root

2. Conconsa

3. Burdock root

4. Yellow dock

5. Marula

6. Lily of the valley

7. Irish Sea moss

How to Use the Revitalizing Herbs Above to Revitalize the Body System After Cleansing for the Treatment of Anemia?

To revitalize the body system after cleansing the body

system for anemia, you will need to focus on purifying the blood, enhancing blood circulation, supporting liver function, aiding iron absorption, etc.

To achieve this, you will need to know the following:

1. Understand the revitalizing herbal combination for anemia

2. How to prepare and administer the herbs

3. The best time to consume the herbs, its storage, and how they can be warmed.

Understand the Revitalizing Herbal Combination for Anemia

1. Purifies blood and enhances blood circulation: Herbal teas made with sarsaparilla root, burdock root, and lily of the valley help to purify the blood, and boost blood circulation. Lily of the Valley also helps support cardiovascular health.

2. Enhances absorption of iron and the immune

system: Herbal teas made with sarsaparilla root, yellow dock root, and marula fruit and seeds help support iron absorption, boost the immune system, and contain some antioxidant properties that help to soothe anemia. Finally, the yellow dock root supports liver functions.

3. Essential minerals and aid revitalization: Herbal teas made with Irish Sea moss and marula fruit or seed helps supply the body with the essential nutrients it needs, and it is very helpful in replenishing the body.

How to Prepare and Administer the Revitalizing Herbal Teas to Revitalize the Body System After Cleansing for Anemia?

To prepare and administer the revitalizing herbs to revitalize the body system after cleansing for Anemia, you will need the following ingredients:

1. 1 tbsp of Sarsaparilla root

2. 1 tbsp of Conconsa bark/root

3. 1 tbsp of Burdock root

4. 1 tbsp of Yellow dock root

5. 1 tbsp of Marula fruit and seeds

6. 1 tbsp of Lily of the Valley flowers

7. 1 tbsp of Irish sea moss gel

The instructions are:

1. Get a clean pot, measure 6-8 cups of water or 48-64 ounces of water, and boil it

2. Once the water is boiling, add the sarsaparilla root, Conconsa bark/root, yellow dock root, and burdock root. Reduce the heat and allow it to simmer for at least 30 minutes.

3. Add marula fruit and lily of the valley flowers and allow it to simmer for another 10-15 minutes before turning off the heat

4. Get a fine mesh, or cheesecloth and strain the tea into a cup or jar to remove the herbal extract.

5. While the tea is still warm, add the Irish Sea moss gel and stir it properly until it's completely dissolved.

Administration of the tea

Start by drinking 1 cup per day for the first three days of your revitalization, before increasing it to 2 cups daily. That is 1/2 cup in the morning and 1/2 cup at night. When you increase your consumption, you can do, 1 cup in the morning and the other 1 cup in the evening to help replenish the body's mineral stores, enhance blood health, and support iron absorption.

Storage and reheating are the same as other herbal teas.

CHAPTER SEVENTEEN
Herbal Remedy for Immune and Respiratory Disorders
The Cleansing Herbs for Boosting of Immune System and the Treatment of Respiratory Disorders.

The cleansing herbs boost the immune and respiratory systems and treat and prevent respiratory system disorders such as asthma, COPD, emphysema, bronchitis, etc. are:

1. Blue Vervain

2. Bugleweed

3. Cablote

4. Cordoncillo negro

5. Elderberry

6. Eucalyptus

7. Guaco

8. Linden

9. Mullein

How to Cleanse the Body System Using the Cleansing Herbs Above to Boost the Immune System and Treat the Respiratory System?

To do a detox to boost the immune system and treat respiratory system disorders, you will need to know the following key things:

1. Understanding the cleansing herbal combination to boost the immune system and treat respiratory system disorders.

2. How to prepare and administer the cleansing herbs.

3. The storage, warming, and best time to consume the cleansing herbs.

Understanding Cleansing Herbal Combination to Boost the Immune System and Treat Respiratory System Disorders

1. Reduction of inflammation and congestion: Herbal teas made with blue vervain, mullein, eucalyptus, cablote, and guaco helps to soothe the lungs and respiratory discomfort, reduce inflammation, and clear mucus from the airways, which eases congestion.

2. Boost respiratory and immune system: Herbal teas made with Bugleweed, Cordoncillo Negro, and elderberry help to boost immunity and support immune and respiratory health.

3. Ease respiratory disorders with its antioxidant, anti-inflammation, and antimicrobial properties Herbal teas made with mullein, linden, guaco, elderberry, and cordoncillo negro help to treat respiratory disorders, reduce respiratory inflammation, and relieve chronic respiratory

disorders.

How to Prepare and Administer the Cleansing Herbal Teas to Boost the Immune System and Treat Respiratory System Disorders?

To prepare and administer the herbal cleansing tea to boost the immune system and treat respiratory system disorders, you will need the following ingredients:

1. 1 tbsp of Blue Vervain leaves flowers, and stems

2. 1 tbsp of Bugleweed aerial parts

3. 1 tbsp of Cablote leaves/stems

4. 1 tbsp of Cordoncillo negro leaves

5. 1 tbsp of Elderberry

6. 1 tbsp of Eucalyptus leaves

7. 1 tbsp of Guaco leaves

8. 1 tbsp of Linden flowers and bracts

9. 1 tbsp of mullein

The Instructions are:

1. Get a clean pot, measure 6-8 cups of water or 48-64 ounces of water, and boil it

2. Once the water is boiling, add Blue Vervain leaves, flowers, and stems, Bugleweed aerial parts, Cablote leaves/stems, and elderberry. Reduce the heat and allow it to simmer for at least 20 minutes.

3. Add Cordoncillo negro leaves, Eucalyptus leaves, Guaco leaves, Linden flowers and bracts, and mullein, and allow it to simmer for an additional 10-15 minutes before turning off the heat.

4. Get a fine mesh, or cheesecloth and strain the herbal tea into a cup or jar to remove the herbal extract.

Administration of the tea

Start by drinking 1 cup per day. Monitor your tolerance level for the first 3 days before you decide to increase your intake to 2 cups per day.

The best time to take this herbal tea is in the morning before breakfast and at night before going to bed. The storage and reheating of the herbal teas are the same.

Don't forget to drink at least a gallon of spring water daily as you desire a fruitful result and your labor will not be in vain in Jesus's name, amen.

The Revitalizing Herbs for the Boosting of the Respiratory and Immune System and the Treatment of the Respiratory Disorders

The revitalizing herbs for boosting the immune and respiratory system and treating and preventing respiratory system disorders such as asthma, COPD, Emphysema, Bronchitis, etc. are:

1. Sarsaparilla root

2. Irish Sea moss

3. Blue Vervain

4. Bugleweed

5. Liden

How to Use the Revitalizing Herbs Above to Revitalize the Body System After Cleansing for Respiratory System Disorder?

To revitalize the body system after cleansing the body system for respiratory system disorders, you will need to know the following:

1. Understand the revitalizing herbal combination for respiratory system disorders.

2. How to prepare and administer the herbs

3. The best time to consume the herbs, its storage, and how they can be warmed.

Understand the Revitalizing Herbal Combination for Respiratory System Disorders

All the herbs are very rich in soothing respiratory system disorders, boosting the immune system, supporting respiratory health, calming, supporting immune and respiratory function, purifying the blood, and are rich with minerals and nutrients that soothe respiratory tissue and nourish the respiratory system.

How to Prepare and Administer Revitalizing Herbal Teas to Revitalize the Body System After Cleansing for Respiratory Disorders?

To prepare and administer the revitalizing herbs to revitalize the body system after cleansing for respiratory disorders, you will need the following ingredients:

1. 1 tbsp Sarsaparilla root

2. 1 tbsp Irish Sea Moss gel

3. 1 tbsp Vervain leaves, flowers, and stems

4. 1 tbsp Bugleweed aerial parts

5. 1 tbsp Linden flowers and bracts

The instructions are:

1. Get a clean pot, measure 4-5 cups of water or 32-40 ounces of water, and boil it

2. Once the water is boiling, add the sarsaparilla root, reduce the heat and allow it to simmer for at least 20 minutes.

3. Add blue vervain, and bugleweed, and allow it to simmer for another 10 minutes.

4. Add the linden and allow it to simmer for another 5-10 minutes before turning off the heat.

5. Use a strainer, fine mesh, or cheesecloth to strain the tea into a cup or jar to remove the herbal extract.

6. While the tea is still warm, add the Irish Sea moss gel and stir it properly until it is completely dissolved.

Administration of the tea

Start by drinking 1 cup per day for the first three days of your revitalization before increasing it to 2 cups daily once you notice that your system tolerates the herbal teas. That is 1/2 cup in the morning and 1/2 cup at night. When you increase your consumption, you can do, 1 cup in the morning and the other 1 cup in the evening to help replenish the body's minerals, enhance energy and blood health, calm, support the respiratory system health, and in the evening to encourage relaxation.

Storage and reheating are the same as other herbal teas.

There must be a change in diet, and you must always eat the following foods:

1. Brazil nut

2. Kale

3. Mushrooms

CHAPTER EIGHTEEN
Tips to Stay Healthy, and Longevity
What is the Human Anatomy, According to Dr. Sebi?

According to Dr. Sebi, human anatomy is built on a natural balance with specific nutritional needs. Based on his beliefs, for a healthy life, one needs to focus on understanding the body's design and why diseases arise whenever one deviates from the natural diet and environment. Unlike what other doctors regard as human anatomy, Dr. Sebi views the human anatomy differently as he sees it as an intricate system with an innate ability to heal itself if it is properly nourished. To him, the body's organs, tissues, and cells are all interconnected and rely on a consistent supply of natural, plant-based nutrients to function excellently. The human anatomy thrives in an alkaline environment, where viruses, bacteria, fungi, etc. cannot survive or even multiply.

However, Dr. Sebi classified their human anatomy into:

1. Cellular Health

2. Alkaline Blood:

3. Nutrient Absorption

4. Organs of Elimination

1. Cellular Health: According to Dr. Sebi, every aspect of the human anatomy, from the cell to organs to tissues to the systems relies on the health of each cell. The body that has healthy cells will function excellently because a cell is the foundation of the biological body, which is made up of the lungs, kidneys, heart, etc., that make up the system like the female reproductive system, male reproductive system, immune system, digestive system, mental clarity, and energy levels.

2. Alkaline Blood: To the late doctor, it is important to maintain an alkaline pH, which he argued that, naturally, the blood should be slightly alkaline (7.3-7.4 pH). This is to prevent diseases that can attack the blood and support cellular health.

3. Nutrient Absorption: According to the late doctor, for the human body to stay healthy, the body needs minerals from natural sources to sustain itself. This is why the bodies absorb nutrients best from alkaline-based plants that are rich in alkaline-forming properties and high in bioavailable minerals.

4. Organs of Elimination: To the late doctor, organs such as the lung, kidney, liver, and colon must be slightly alkaline as they are responsible for eliminating waste and toxins. When these organs are compromised, toxins accumulate, and

the body relapses to illness.

What Makes Humans Fall Sick, According to Dr. Sebi?

According to Dr. Sebi, disease originates from two primary factors, which are:

1. An acidic environment

2. Mucus buildup.

The doctor argued that most diseases the human body suffers from stem from these causes, which he regards as the root causes of illness. Once any of the body's organs or systems are compromised, it can lead to inflammation, poor circulation, and toxic buildup.

According to the doctor, excess mucus in the body is the root of most illnesses. He stated that mucus is the body's response to toxins and acidity. For example, if the respiratory tract is compromised with mucus, it could lead to respiratory disorders such as Asthma or bronchitis. The compromising of the reproductive

---

system with mucus will lead to infertility, low sperm count, premature ejaculation, etc. The compromising of the tissue with mucous can lead to a reduction in oxygen and nutrient flow, and disrupt cellular communication, leading to disease. To him, there is only one disease and one cure, and the disease is the accumulation of mucus in the body.

To rid the body of this excess mucus through an alkaline diet will help the body reverse these issues. Once the body is no longer alkaline but too acidic, it becomes a breeding ground for disease. An acidic environment weakens the immune system and creates inflammation, contributing to a variety of diseases such as diabetes, high blood pressure, arthritis, heart disease, etc.

Acidity also makes the body vulnerable to pathogens, as bacteria, viruses, and fungi thrive in an acidic setting.

The doctor also argued that processed foods,

unnatural sugars, artificial additives, and preservatives disrupt cellular health and clog the body's natural detox pathways thereby giving room to the body to become acidic weakening the organs, (liver and kidneys) thereby making the body a disease enabling environment.

Genetically modified foods, heavily processed foods, or non-alkaline foods contribute to cellular decay, and over time, the cumulative effects of these toxins lead to chronic diseases.

The human body needs natural, alkaline foods such as fruits, vegetables, herbs, and certain grains to stay healthy. The absensibility of alkaline diets in the body means the body lacks essential nutrients and minerals for the cellular to stay healthy, energize, and support immune function.

The minerals in Plant-alkaline foods support all body functions, from brain activity to digestion, too respiratory to reproductive, and the deficiency in these nutrients leads to a weakened immunity and poor organ function leading to diseases.

According to Dr. Sebi, the human digestive system is built to process natural foods, and if we can stick to eating only natural food, the digestive system cannot be compromised and no one will be sick, but the reverse is the case. This is why people are suffering from cellular health, immune deficiency, autoimmune diseases, cancer, etc., as their bodies cannot effectively use nutrients from unnatural or acidic foods.

How Do I Maintain An Alkalinity for Health and Longevity

According to the late doctor, adopting an alkaline diet rich in plant-based foods helps to maintain the original natural alkaline state that the body is supposed to maintain, and by avoiding processed, acidic foods and focusing on nutrient-dense, whole foods, the body can stay balanced and free from diseases. If you follow this approach, you are certain to live a life of longevity, and the body's self-healing abilities will be enhanced and align with the body's original, alkaline nature.

For any enquiries, kindly subscribe to our YouTube channel where we drop health update at least once in a week and you can ask any questions there.

YouTube:

https://m.youtube.com/@backtoedenwithclem

X: http://x.com/HerbalR67752

Ig:

https://www.instagram.com/backtoedenwithclem/

Facebook:

https://www.facebook.com/profile.php?id=6156817 3853698&name=xhp_nt_fb_action_open_user

Please like and follow us on all our social media handles. Thank you.

Chat on WhatsApp with +234 807 074 4963

About the Author

Clement Jacob is a passionate advocate for natural health and wellness, dedicated to exploring alternative approaches to self-healing. With a deep understanding of Dr. Sebi's TWO STEPS OF HEALING METHODOLOGY with alkaline diets and spring water. Clement offers a practical guide for those interested in managing health conditions naturally. His latest book, "Dr. sebi's approved encyclopedia for alkaline herbal remedies," provides insights into natural methods for supporting health and addressing conditions like ERECTILE DYSFUNCTION, INFERTILITY, high blood pressure, diabetes, skin diseases, and more.

Other books written by Clement Jacob that can be found on Amazon include:

Dr. Sebi: 100% Natural Erectile Dysfunction Treatment! Dr. Sebi: 100% Natural Remedy 4 Female Reproductive System Disorders!

Dr. Sebi: 100% Natural Remedy 4 Respiratory Disorders,

etc.

Made in United States
North Haven, CT
01 July 2025